The Nursing Assistant's Handbook

By Hartman Publishing, Inc.

Credits

MANAGING EDITOR
Susan Alvare

DESIGN/ILLUSTRATOR
Thaddeus Castillo

COMPOSITION
Susan Alvare

PROOFREADER
Celia McIntire

Notice to Readers

Though the guidelines and procedures contained in this text are based on consultations with healthcare professionals, they should not be considered absolute recommendations. The instructor and readers should follow employer, local, state, and federal guidelines concerning healthcare practices. These guidelines change, and it is the reader's responsibility to be aware of these changes and of the policies and procedures of her or his healthcare facility. The publisher, author, editors, and reviewers cannot accept any responsibility for errors or omissions or for any consequences from application of the information in this book and make no warranty, expressed or implied, with respect to the contents of the book. The Publisher does not warrant or guarantee any of the products described herein or perform any analysis in connection with any of the product information contained herein.

Copyright Information

Welcome to the Workbook!

This book is designed to help you review what you have learned from reading your textbook. For this reason, the workbook is organized around learning objectives, just like your textbook and even your instructor's teaching material. By including the learning objectives, it makes it easier for you to go back and reread a section if you need to refresh your memory.

We have provided checklists for the procedures close to the end of the workbook. There is also a practice exam for the certification test at the end of the workbook. The answers to the workbook exercises are in your instructor's teaching guide.

Happy Learning!

ONE

Long-Term Care and the Nursing Assistant's Role

Unit 1. Compare long-term care to other healthcare settings

Matching.

Write the letter of the correct definition beside each term listed below.

a. Care provided in a person's home.

b. Care performed in hospitals for temporary, but serious, illnesses or injuries.

c. Care performed by a specially-trained therapist to restore or improve function after an illness or injury.

d. Short-term care usually provided for less than 24-hours for persons who have had treatments or surgery.

e. Care provided for persons who need some daily assistance but do not need skilled care.

f. Care for persons who are dying and their families.

g. Persons who live in nursing homes.

h. Care in a hospital or nursing home for persons who need more observation and daily care than a long-term care facility can offer.

i. Twenty-four hour care and assistance for long-term conditions. Other terms for this type of care include nursing home or extended care facility.

j. Conditions that last a long period of time.

1. __D__ Acute care

2. __E__ Assisted living

3. __A__ Home care

4. __F__ Hospice

5. __B__ Outpatient care

6. __H__ Rehabilitation

7. __C__ Chronic

8. __I__ Subacute care

9. __J__ Long-term care

10. __G__ Residents

Unit 2: Describe a typical long-term care facility

True or False.

Mark each statement with either a "T" for true or "F" for false.

1. __F__ LTC facilities do not have dementia units.

2. __T__ When specialized care is offered in a LTC facility, employees need special training.

3. __F T__ Subacute care is never offered in a LTC facility.

4. __T__ Nonprofit organizations can own LTC facilities.

Unit 3: Explain Medicare and Medicaid

Fill in the Blank.

Write the correct answer in the blanks below.

1. CMS runs two national healthcare programs: Medicare & Medicaid.

Name: _____

2. Medicare is a health insurance program for people over ___65___ years old. It also covers people who are _disabled & unable to work_.

3. Medicare and Medicaid both help pay for _Health care_ and _Health insurance_ for millions of Americans.

4. The Centers for Medicare & Medicaid Services (CMS) was formerly called the _Health Care Finance Administration_.

5. Medicaid is a medical assistance program for _low-income_ people.

6. Medicare and Medicaid pay long-term care facilities a _fixed_ amount for services for residents.

Unit 4: Describe the role of the nursing assistant

Short Answer.

1. What are some things you think you'll like most about being a nursing assistant?

   Helping take care of people with their every day needs

2. Why is a nursing assistant one of the most important members of the health-care team?

   This one hands on with the patients or residents. Their vital signs are also very important, and you would be taking their vitals.

Unit 5: Describe the care team and the chain of command

Crossword.

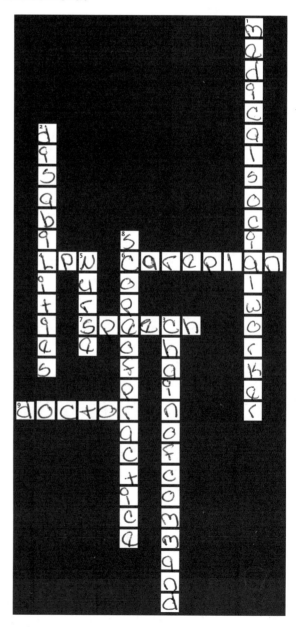

Clues:

Across

4. Person who passes medications and performs treatments

   LPN

6. Developed for each resident to achieve certain goals

   care plan

7. Type of therapist who evaluates a person's ability to swallow food and drink

   speech

9. Person who diagnoses disease or disability and prescribes treatment

   doctor

Down

1. Helps a resident locate clothing if her family lives far away

   medical social worker

2. An occupational therapist helps residents learn to compensate for these.

   disabilities

3. Guarantees that your residents get proper health care

   chain of command

5. One role of this person is to develop a nursing assistant care plan for each resident.

   nurse

8. Only doing things you are allowed to do and doing them correctly

   scope of practice

Labeling.

Fill in the blanks of the chain of command with members of the healthcare team. Some have already been filled in for you.

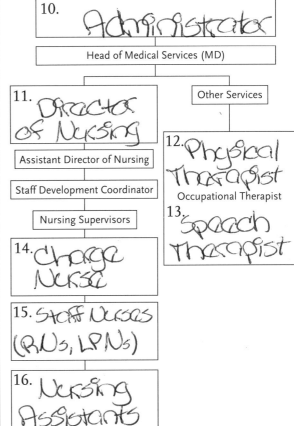

10. *Administrator*

Head of Medical Services (MD)

11. *Director of Nursing*

Assistant Director of Nursing

Staff Development Coordinator

Nursing Supervisors

14. *Charge Nurse*

15. *Staff Nurses (RNs, LPNs)*

16. *Nursing Assistants*

Other Services

12. *Physical Therapist*

Occupational Therapist

13. *Speech Therapist*

True or False.

Mark each statement with either a "T" for true or "F" for false.

17. *F* The purpose of the care plan is to give suggestions for care, which the nursing assistant can choose whether to follow or not.

18. *T* Activities that are not listed on the care plan should not be performed without permission from the nurse.

Name: _____

Unit 6: Define policies, procedures, and professionalism

Multiple Choice.

Circle the correct response.

1. Examples of common policies at long-term care facilities include all EXCEPT one of the following:
   a. Keeping all information confidential
   b. Following the resident's plan of care
   c. Discussing troubles at home with your resident
   d. Performing only tasks that are included in your job description

2. Which of the following is NOT an example of having a professional relationship with a resident?
   a. Asking your resident "Can you give me a few minutes? I've just had a fight with my boyfriend."
   b. Asking, "Mr. Gomez, would you mind if I entered your room?"
   c. Listening to Ms. Petrie while she talks about a loved one's death.
   d. Explaining to Mrs. Olsen about the bath you are going to give her.

3. Which of the following is an example of compassionate behavior?
   a. Making fun of Mrs. Klepstein's baggy sweater.
   b. Making sure that other people cannot see your resident while you are helping her dress.
   c. Telling other nursing assistants about a resident who cried in front of you.
   d. Laughing when a resident tells you she thinks she is very sick.

4. Being respectful towards a resident includes:
   a. Telling her that you do not like the cross she wears around her neck

   b. Deciding on your own to rearrange his room
   c. Mentioning to her that she needs a haircut
   d. Calling him by the name he wishes to be called

Mark an "X" by all examples of a professional relationship with an employer.

5. __X__ maintaining a positive attitude

6. __X__ completing duties efficiently

7. _____ deciding for yourself when you should and should not follow policies and procedures

8. __X__ always documenting and reporting carefully and correctly

9. __X__ keeping problems you have with residents a secret

10. _____ never asking questions when you do not know or understand something

11. __X__ taking directions or criticism without getting upset

12. __X__ being clean and neatly dressed

13. _____ being late for work

14. _____ forgetting to call in if you cannot make it to work

15. __X__ following the chain of command

16. __X__ participating in education programs offered

17. __X__ being a positive role model for your facility at all times

Unit 7: List examples of legal and ethical behavior and explain residents' rights

Case Studies.

Read the following sentences and answer the question.

Matt, a new nursing assistant, tells a resident that she has to wear the flowered shirt he picked out for her.

1. Which residents' right does this violate?

Quality of Life

Margaret, a nursing assistant, tells her best friend, "Ms. Picadilly's cancer is getting worse. I heard her moaning all night last night."

2. Which residents' right does this violate?

Privicy and confidentiality

Harry, a nursing assistant, is taking vital signs on his resident when the resident's family arrives. He tells them, "You'll have to come back another day. I'm busy with her right now."

3. Which residents' right does this violate?

Yvonne, a nursing assistant, is going off duty. Leaving Ms. Rice's room, she notices a pretty necklace. She decides to borrow it for

the night, promising to herself to return it tomorrow. She knows Ms. Robins has Alzheimer's and won't notice that it is gone anyway.

4. Which residents' right does this violate?

Security of possessions

Mrs. Holland is a confused resident. When she can't find her purse, she yells at her nursing assistant, "What did you do with my purse? I know you stole it." Jake, her nursing assistant, responds, "Shut up, crazy old coot. I didn't take anything!"

5. Which residents' right does this violate?

Voice complaints

You are the nursing assistant for a resident who is paralyzed on her right side from a recent stroke. Some of her family members are visiting and one of them turns to you and says in a loud voice, "She looks so stupid with half of her face drooping down like that. Isn't there something you can do to fix that?"

6. What kind of abuse is this?
    a. physical abuse
    b. psychological abuse
    c. invasion of privacy
    d. none of the above

Name: _____

You see a nursing assistant slap a resident with dementia on the hand because she is yelling and refusing to let the nursing assistant bathe her.

7. What kind of abuse is this?

  (a.) physical abuse

  b. psychological abuse

  c. neglect

  d. domestic violence

8. If you suspect an elderly resident is being abused, you must:

  a. ask another resident if he thinks that person is being abused

  b. ask your family and friends for advice

  (c.) report it to your supervisor and let him/her handle it from there

  d. do nothing since someone has probably already reported it

9. If a resident refuses to take a bath, you should:

  a. offer her a prize if she will take the bath

  (b.) respect her wishes, but report it to the nurse

  c. tell her you are going to leave if she does not bathe

  d. force her to take the bath

Unit 8: Explain legal aspects of the resident's medical record

Short Answer.

1. List the four reasons why careful documentation is important.

- It is the only way to guarantee clear & complete communication between all the members of the care team.

- can be used as legal records.

- protects you & your employer.

- provides an up-to-date record of your resident.

2. Why should you write your notes immediately after giving care?

This helps you remember important details

TWO

Foundations of Resident Care

Unit 1: Understand the importance of verbal and written communications

Multiple Choice.

Circle the letter of the answer that best completes the statement or answers the question.

1. Which of the following is an example of verbal communication?

   (a.) telling a joke

   b. laughing at a joke

2. Which of the following is an example of nonverbal communication?

   a. asking for a glass of water

   (b.) pointing to a glass of water

3. Types of verbal communication include:

   a. writing

   b. nodding your head

   c. speaking

   (d) both a and c

4. Types of nonverbal communication include:

   a. speaking

   (b.) facial expressions

   c. the way you say something

   (d.) none of the above

5. Which of the following is an example of a confusing or conflicting message (saying one thing and meaning another)?

   a. Mr. Carter smiles happily and tells you he is excited because his daughter is coming to visit.

   (b.) Mrs. Sanchez looks like she is in pain. When you ask her about it, she tells you that her back has been bothering her lately.

   (c.) Ms. Jones agrees with you when you say it is a nice day, but she looks angry.

   d. Mr. Wilson won't watch his favorite TV show. He says he feels a little depressed.

Labeling.

Looking at the diagram, list examples of observations using each sense.

6. Smell:

   residents body or breath odor.

7. Sight:

   change in appearance rashes, redness, paleness, swelling.

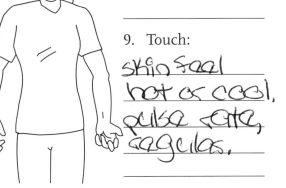

8. Hearing:

   thics words tone & breathing.

9. Touch:

   skin feel hot or cool, pulse rate, regular.

Name: _____

Short Answer.

For each of the following, decide whether it is an objective observation (you can see, hear, smell, or touch it) or subjective observation (the resident must tell you about it). Write "O" for objective and "S" for subjective.

10. __O__ Skin rash

11. __O__ Crying

12. __O__ Rapid pulse

13. __S__ Headache

14. __S__ Nausea

15. __O__ Vomiting

16. __O__ Swelling

17. __O__ Cloudy urine

18. __S__ Depression

19. __O__ Redness

20. __O__ Fever

21. __S__ Dizziness

22. __O__ Noisy breathing

23. __S__ Chest pain

24. __S__ Toothache

25. __O__ Coughing

26. __S__ Painful breathing

27. __O__ Fruity breath

28. __S__ Itching

Unit 2: Describe barriers to communication

Word Search.

Complete each of the following sentences and find your answers in the word search.

1. Do not offer your personal
   __opinion__
   to the resident or give
   __advice__ .

2. __slang__ words or expressions may not be understood and are unprofessional.

3. __cliches__ are phrases that don't really mean anything.

4. Be __patient__ with a resident who is difficult to understand.

5. If a resident does not hear you or does not understand you, speak more __slowly__ .

6. If a resident does not understand you, speak in __simple__ , everyday words.

7. Each person's background, values, and __language__ affect communication.

s	t	o	v	a	f	p	o	f	w	z	a	s	z
l	y	v	o	s	b	s	w	c	z	d	l	o	m
a	c	o	y	z	i	z	i	l	v	o	g	m	h
n	i	l	o	x	g	g	a	i	w	d	w	k	t
g	r	o	i	n	d	n	c	l	s	a	p	h	s
s	u	c	y	c	g	e	y	e	u	h	l	q	d
e	o	p	k	u	h	o	f	l	n	l	j	f	o
k	p	j	a	h	e	e	p	x	e	w	v	y
q	w	g	f	r	u	z	s	i	l	h	g	z	f
h	e	q	k	x	q	i	t	n	p	s	o	y
k	r	n	t	x	f	q	g	g	d	i	m	e	l
r	x	n	x	u	o	l	x	e	h	f	o	i	o
f	p	u	h	u	s	g	k	l	f	z	u	n	s
x	f	x	n	u	b	s	t	n	e	i	t	a	p

Unit 3: List guidelines for communicating with residents with special needs

Nursing assistant Josh Lucas is about to provide care for hearing-impaired resident Mrs. Castillo. She is standing at the window looking out at the gardens. He enters her room and asks if she would like her hair shampooed. She doesn't answer. He taps her on the back, and she jumps. He yells, "I said, would you like to have your hair shampooed now?"

Name: _____
13

1. What would have been a correct way for Josh to communicate with Mrs. Castillo?

Come in and tap her shoulder or called her name so she could see him, then asked again face to face.

Not to of said that and just forgot about it & talk normal, simple words, even if they don't talk back.

Vision-impaired resident Ms. Crawford is being helped into a fellow resident's room for a visit. Nursing assistant Virginia Davies assists her to the door and says, "See you later, Ms. Crawford. I'll be back in about an hour to help you return to your room." Ms. Crawford enters the room, walks into a chair and almost falls over.

2. What would have been a correct way for Virginia to communicate with Ms. Crawford?

to walk her over to where she would be safe or sit her down.

Kelley, a nursing assistant, is taking care of a mentally ill resident who is very withdrawn. Kelley moves around the room picking up clutter and speaking to her resident in a bored tone: "How are we doing today, Mrs. Rogers? Are we going to start talking to Kelley today, or are we going to be quiet like we were yesterday?"

3. What would have been a correct way for Kelley to communicate with Mrs. Rogers?

Resident Joe Morteno has dementia and can be aggressive at times. On this particular day he lashes out at nursing assistant Serena Jones. "Why are you so stupid? You never understand what I really need," he yells. Serena replies, "I'm not stupid. You're the one who is stupid."

4. What would have been a correct way for Serena to communicate with Mr. Morteno?

She shouldn't have talked back and should have told the supervisor.

Unit 4: Identify ways to promote safety and handle non-medical emergencies

Short Answer.

1. Looking at the illustration on the next page, which picture shows the correct way to lift objects? Why is it correct?

B, because he's bent at the knees and it won't strain his back.

Name: _____

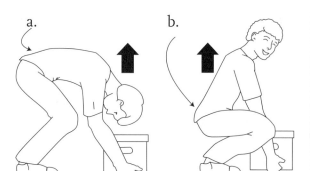

a.   b.

2. Why should you arrange a signal, such as counting to three, when you are moving a resident?

So you both can work together at the same time.

True or False.

Mark each statement with either a "T" for true or "F" for false.

3. __T__ By applying the principles of good body mechanics to your work, you can avoid injury and save energy.

4. __T__ To guard against choking, residents should eat sitting as upright as possible.

5. __F__ To lift a heavy object from the floor, you must first place your feet together and keep your knees straight.

6. __T__ The muscles of the thighs, upper arms, and shoulders are not as strong as the muscles in the back.

7. __F__ Thickened liquids are harder to swallow.

8. __T__ To help guard against falls, clear all walkways of clutter, throw rugs, and cords.

9. __T__ A wide base of support and a low center of gravity means the feet are apart and the knees are bent.

10. __T__ When moving an object, pivot your feet instead of twisting at the waist.

11. __F__ It is a good idea to hold an object away from your body, because this helps you balance the weight more evenly.

12. __T__ Never try to catch a falling resident as you could seriously injure yourself and/or the resident.

13. __F__ Bending from the waist allows you to use the big muscles in your legs and hips rather than the smaller muscles in your back.

14. __T__ Always check water temperature with a water thermometer or on your wrist before using it.

15. __T__ Call lights that are not left within a resident's reach can raise the risk for falls.

16. __F__ If your clothing catches fire, run as fast as you can to the nearest exit.

Fill in the meanings of the following two acronyms.

17. To operate a fire extinguisher:

P pull the pin

A aim at the base of the fire

S squeeze handle

S sweep back & forth

18. In case of a fire:

R _remove resident_
from danger

A _activate alarm_

_____

C _contain fire as_
possible

E _extinguish_

_____

Labeling.

Looking at the illustration below, fill in the three parts of the ABC's of good body mechanics.

19. _alignment_

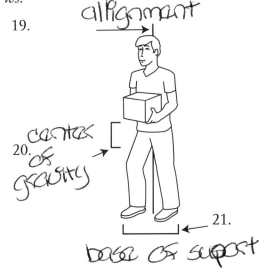

20. _center of gravity_

21. _base of support_

Unit 5: Demonstrate how to recognize and respond to medical emergencies

Short Answer.

1. When you come upon an emergency situation, what two important steps should you follow?

you should assess the situation & assess the victim

Matching.

Write the letter of the correct definition beside each term listed on the following page.

a. Signs of this include pale or bluish skin, staring, increased pulse and respiration rate, decreased blood pressure, and extreme thirst.

b. Signs of this include severe pain in the chest, anxiety, and a feeling of indigestion.

c. This artery in the neck will help you check for a person's pulse.

d. It is called this when something is blocking the tube through which air enters the lungs.

e. Give abdominal thrusts until the object is pushed out or the person loses consciousness.

f. You must apply firm pressure on the wound with a pad or clean cloth when this occurs.

g. If a person is sitting, have her bend forward and place her head between her knees.

h. Signs of this include loss of consciousness, loss of bowel and bladder control, and use of inappropriate words.

i. Do not try to force anything in a person's mouth, including your hands, when this is happening.

j. Two ways to check for this include looking for the chest to rise and fall and putting your ear near the person's nose and mouth.

k. If there is no breathing, open the mouth and try to sweep the mouth with your finger to remove the blockage.

l. Sweet or fruity breath is a symptom.

m. This can result from either too much insulin or too little food.

Name: _____

2. __D__ heart attack

3. __S__ bleeding

4. __C__ carotid artery

5. __e__ performing the Heimlich maneuver for the conscious person

6. __a__ shock

7. __g__ fainting

8. __d__ obstructed airway

9. __h__ stroke

10. __i__ seizure

11. __L__ diabetic coma

12. __m__ insulin shock

13. __j__ breathing

14. __k__ performing the Heimlich maneuver for the unconscious person

Unit 6: Describe and demonstrate infection control practices

Multiple Choice.

Circle the letter of the answer that best completes the statement or answers the question.

1. The following are necessary links in the chain of infection. By wearing gloves, which link is broken and thus prevents the spread of disease?

   a. reservoir (place where the pathogen lives and grows)

   b. mode of transmission (a way for the disease to spread)

   c. susceptible host (person who is likely to get the disease)

   d. none of the above

2. The following are necessary links in the chain of infection. By getting a vaccination shot for Hepatitis B, which link will be affected and thus prevent you from getting Hepatitis B?

   a. reservoir (place where the pathogen lives and grows)

   b. mode of transmission (a way for the disease to spread)

   c. susceptible host (person who is likely to get the disease)

   d. none of the above

3. Standard Precautions should be practiced:

   a. only on people who look like they have a bloodborne disease

   b. on every single person in your care

   c. only on people who request that you follow them

   d. none of the above

4. Standard Precautions include the following measures:

   a. Washing your hands before putting on and after removing gloves

   b. Wearing gloves if there is a possibility you will come into contact with blood, body fluids, mucous membranes, or broken skin

   c. Touching body fluids with your bare hands

   d. a and b

5. The single most important thing you can do to prevent the spread of disease is to:

   a. carry dirty linen close to your uniform

   b. never change your gloves

   c. remove gloves before cleaning spills

   d. wash your hands

6. Which of the following is true for Transmission-Based Precautions?

   a. You do not need to practice Standard Precautions if you practice Transmission-Based Precautions.

   b. They are exactly the same as Standard Precautions.

c. They are practiced in addition to Standard Precautions.

d. none of the above

Mark an "X" next to the tasks that require you to wear gloves.

7. _X_ handling body fluids

8. ____ moving a resident's picture

9. _X_ anytime you may touch blood

10. ____ combing a resident's hair

11. _X_ assisting with perineal care

12. _X_ giving a massage to a resident with broken skin on his back

13. _X_ performing mouth care

14. _X_ shaving a resident

Short Answer.

15. What should you always do after touching any body substance, handling contaminated items, or removing gloves?

wash your hands

16. After giving care to a resident, why should you remove your gloves before leaving the room?

so the bacteria doesn't spread anywhere else or contaminate anything else.

17. Why do you think PPE is so important in the healthcare setting?

so you stay clean and don't contaminate.

18. Why is it important to communicate with a resident who is in isolation?

so they know what you are going to do

19. When putting on PPE, what is the correct order?

1st mask & eye shield

2nd gown

3rd gloves

20. When removing PPE, what is the correct order?

1st gloves

2nd gown

3rd mask & eye shield

True or False.

Mark each statement with either a "T" for true or "F" for false.

21. _T_ Mask and eye protection are worn while providing care if there is a chance that a splash or spray may occur.

22. _F_ Airborne precautions are used when a microorganism does not stay suspended in the air.

Name: _____

23. __T__ Laughing and sneezing can generate droplets.

24. __T__ Employers offer a free vaccine for Hepatitis B.

25. __T__ Tuberculosis is an example of an airborne disease.

26. __F__ When handling soiled linens, keep them close to your uniform.

27. __T__ Contact precautions include not touching an infected surface without wearing gloves.

THREE

Understanding Your Residents

Unit 1: Explain why promoting independence and self-care is important

Word Search.

Complete each of the following sentences and find your answers in the word search.

o	k	w	s	e	c	n	e	d	n	e	p	e	d
z	i	h	t	g	z	e	g	s	k	c	i	v	z
l	b	n	k	v	x	z	o	s	a	h	d	p	b
p	h	r	d	g	c	k	a	c	t	n	d	e	n
s	p	n	h	e	s	t	t	q	q	k	z	s	b
m	o	o	w	v	p	i	s	i	i	l	i	i	m
m	c	d	u	z	v	e	h	v	s	z	n	e	r
m	d	h	z	i	y	r	n	u	w	y	a	c	g
x	o	h	t	q	y	h	v	d	z	m	w	p	t
a	r	i	n	s	w	a	s	m	e	x	g	s	g
a	e	c	w	b	d	z	a	l	i	n	x	c	s
s	p	v	p	r	h	d	t	q	i	p	c	t	v
e	m	p	a	t	h	y	i	a	h	e	g	e	g
t	e	q	i	x	x	e	r	a	c	f	l	e	s

1. A loss of ___*independence*___ is very difficult for a person to deal with.

2. Allow and encourage a resident to do a ___*task*___ for himself even if it's easier for you to do it.

3. ___*empathy*___ is the ability to share feelings with another person by putting yourself in her shoes.

4. ___*activities*___ of daily living (ADLs) are personal care tasks done every day to care for yourself.

5. Encourage ___*resident*___ regardless of how long it takes or how poorly he is able to do it.

6. A loss of independence can cause increased ___*dependence*___.

Read the following paragraph and answer the question below.

Sarah, a nursing assistant, is assisting resident Mrs. Sanchez today. It is time to get Mrs. Sanchez dressed and ready for breakfast. Sarah enters the room without knocking. She doesn't see Mrs. Sanchez. She walks over to the bathroom door and opens it. Mrs. Sanchez is pulling up her underpants. "Hurry up," says Sarah. "We've got to get you dressed."

Sarah chooses and lays out clean clothes. Mrs. Sanchez starts to take off her nightgown but has trouble getting it over her head. Sarah impatiently reaches over and yanks it over her head. "Sit down. It will be faster if I do this." She quickly starts putting a clean shirt on Mrs. Sanchez.

7. List all of the examples of how Sarah did NOT promote privacy, dignity, and independence.

she knock before entering the room, she just opened the bathroom door without seeing the resident, tells her to hurry, doesn't ask what she want to wear, she yanked it over her head.

Name: _____

Short Answer.

8. Write a brief paragraph explaining everything you did this morning before arriving in class. Include things such as bathing, going to the bathroom, applying makeup, brushing your hair, brushing your teeth, walking around your house, etc. Then answer the question below.

_____

_____

_____

_____

_____

_____

_____

_____

_____

_____

9. How would you feel if you were unable to do one or more of these tasks by yourself?

_____

_____

_____

_____

_____

_____

_____

_____

_____

Unit 2: Identify basic human needs

Multiple Choice.

Circle the letter of the answer that best completes the statement or answers the question.

1. Basic physical needs include:
   a. need for self-esteem
   b. food and water
   c. social interaction with others
   d. all of the above

2. If you encounter a resident in a sexual situation, you should:
   a. provide privacy
   b. tell him that what he is doing is wrong
   c. tell another nursing assistant that the resident is disgusting
   d. none of the above

3. Psychosocial needs include the following:
   a. love and affection
   b. feeling safe and secure
   c. accomplishments and self-esteem
   d. all of the above

Mark an "X" next to examples of good ways to assist residents with their spiritual needs.

4. X____ A resident tells you that he cannot drink milk with his hamburger due to his religious beliefs. He asks you for some water instead. You notify the nurse, take the drink away, and bring him some water.

5. ____ A resident tells you she is a Baptist and wants to know when the next Baptist service will be. "A Baptist?" you ask. "Why don't you just attend a Catholic service? One is starting in ten minutes."

6. X____ A resident asks you to read a passage from his Bible. He tells you that it will comfort him. You open the Bible and begin to read.

7. X____ A resident wants to see a rabbi. You report this request to the nurse.

8. _____ You see a Buddha statue in a resident's room. You laugh and tell the resident, "I couldn't keep this thing next to my bed. It would make me laugh too much."

9. __X__ A spiritual leader is visiting with a resident. You quietly leave the room and shut the door.

10. _____ A resident tells you he is Muslim. You begin to explain Christianity to him and ask him to attend a Presbyterian service just to see what it's like.

11. __X__ A resident tells you that she doesn't believe in God. You do believe in God but do not argue with her. You listen quietly as she tells you her reasons.

Labeling.

Fill in the following blanks to complete the types of needs in "Maslow's Hierarchy of Needs."

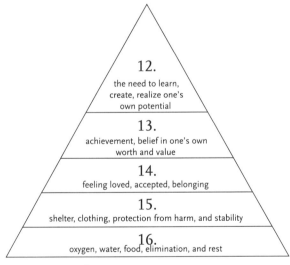

12.
the need to learn, create, realize one's own potential

13.
achievement, belief in one's own worth and value

14.
feeling loved, accepted, belonging

15.
shelter, clothing, protection from harm, and stability

16.
oxygen, water, food, elimination, and rest

12. need for self-actualization
13. need for self-esteem
14. need for love
15. safety & security
16. physical needs

Unit 3: Identify ways to accommodate cultural differences

Crossword.

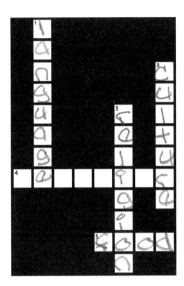

Clues:

Across

4. You can't expect to be treated the same way by all of your residents; you may have to adjust this around each of them.

_____

5. Religious beliefs may include restrictions on this and must be respected.

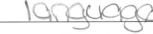
food

Down

1. An interpreter can help you understand this if a resident speaks a different one.

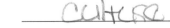
language

2. A system of behaviors people learn from the people with whom they grow up and live

culture

3. When people are ill or dying, this may become especially important.

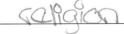
religion

Name: _____

Short Answer.

6. Briefly describe the culture in which you grew up.

_____
_____
_____
_____
_____
_____
_____
_____
_____
_____

Unit 4: Discuss family roles and their significance in health care

Short Answer.

1. List four ways families help residents in long-term care.

- make care decisions
- communicating w/the care team.
- give support & encouragement
- offering assurance

2. What is some important information that family members can contribute about residents?

_____
_____
_____
_____
_____
_____

True or False.

Mark each statement with either a "T" for true or "F" for false.

3. __F__ It is okay to discuss any medical information about a resident with his family members.

4. __T__ A family can be an unmarried couple.

5. __T__ Families play a huge role in most people's lives.

6. __F__ Do not ask a family questions about when a resident likes to eat breakfast.

Unit 5: Describe the stages of human development

Fill in the Blank.

1. Infants develop from the __head__ down.

2. Toddlers learn to __speak__ and control their bladders and bowels.

3. Children in their preschool years begin to learn right from __wrong__.

4. School-age children develop a conscience, morals, and __self-esteem__.

5. __Puberty__ occurs between the ages of 10 to 16 for girls and 12 to 14 for boys.

6. Adolescents are concerned with __body__ image and acceptance by their peers.

7. Young adults may select a __mate__.

8. Generalizations about older adults are often __false__.

Short Answer.

9. In the movies or on television, older peo-

ple are usually portrayed as slow, lonely, helpless, or dependent. However, this is often false. Can you think of a positive portrayal of an older person on television or in a movie? If so, list it here. Briefly describe what you like about the character.

_____

_____

_____

_____

Mark an "X" next to normal changes of aging.

10. _____ depression

11. __X__ drier skin

12. __X__ mild forgetfulness

13. _____ incontinence

14. _____ not eating properly

15. __X__ less efficient heart

16. __X__ more frequent elimination

17. __X__ weaker muscles

Unit 6: Discuss the needs of people with developmental disabilities

Short Answer.

1. List some of the abilities that may be affected by developmental disabilities.

_____

_____

_____

_____

Unit 7: Explain how to care for dying residents

Multiple Choice.

Circle the letter of the answer that best completes the statement or answers the question.

1. Mrs. Levine, a resident, prays about her terminal illness. She promises God that she will make peace with her sister whom she has not seen in 20 years if she is allowed to live. Which stage of dying is Mrs. Levine going through?

    a. denial

    b. anger

    c. bargaining

    d. depression

    e. acceptance

2. A terminally ill resident, Mr. Lucero, begins to yell at Peter, his nursing assistant. He says that he never took good care of him. He blames Peter for a lack of proper care. Peter does not take it personally because he realizes that Mr. Lucero may be going through the _____ stage of dying.

    a. denial

    b. anger

    c. bargaining

    d. depression

    e. acceptance

3. Resident Wilda Scott is dying. Her priest visits her at her request. When he asks her if there is anything he can do to help her get things in order, she tells him she has no idea what he is talking about. Instead she begins to tell him the latest news about her son. Mrs. Scott is experiencing:

    a. denial

    b. anger

    c. bargaining

    d. depression

    e. acceptance

4. A terminally ill resident, John Castillo, visits with his family. He discusses his funeral arrangements with them. He lets them know that he is concerned about

their well-being after he is gone. He says he wants to spend as much time as possible with them before he dies. Mr. Castillo is going through the _____ stage of dying.

a. denial

b. anger

(c.) bargaining

d. depression

e. acceptance

5. A terminally ill resident cries constantly. She doesn't want to talk to anyone. She may be experiencing the _____ stage of dying.

a. denial

b. anger

c. bargaining

(d.) depression

e. acceptance

True or False.

Mark each statement with either a "T" for true or "F" for false.

6. __T__ Listening to a resident who is dying is very important.

7. __F__ All people grieve in the same way.

8. __T__ Hearing is usually the last sense to leave the body.

9. __T__ A person may be incontinent after death.

10. __F__ Skin care is not important for a dying resident.

11. __T__ Keep the room softly lighted for a dying resident.

12. __T__ Blurred vision is a sign of approaching death.

13. __F__ It is important to observe dying residents for signs of pain.

14. __F__ Mouth care should not be given to dying residents.

Unit 8: Define the goals of a hospice program

Short Answer.

1. How are the goals of care different in hospice care than in long-term care?

Hospice is for people who only have 6 months or less & don't take anything to prolong thier life, LTCF

Fill in the Blank.

2. A hospice can be any location where a person who is dying is treated with __dignity__ by caregivers.

3. Residents who are dying also need to feel some __independence__ for as long as possible.

4. In hospice care, the focus is on relieving residents' __pain__ and making them comfortable, rather than on teaching them to care for themselves.

5. Recognize that some persons wish to be __alone__ with their dying loved ones.

6. Be a good __listener__ to a dying resident, and do not feel obligated to respond.

FOUR

Body Systems

Word Search.

Looking at all ten of the body systems, fill in the blanks below, and find your answers in the word search.

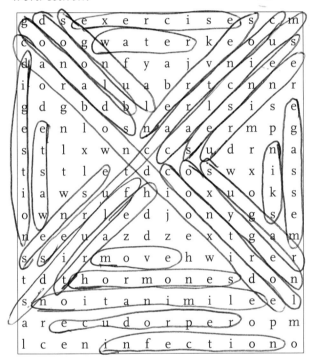

1. The largest organ and system in the body is the ___skin___.

2. Skin prevents the loss of too much ___water___, which is essential to life.

3. The skin is also a ___sense___ organ that feels heat, cold, pain, touch, and pressure.

4. Muscles, bones, ligaments, tendons, and cartilage work together to allow the body to ___move___.

5. ___exercise___ is important for improving and maintaining physical and mental health.

6. ___contractures___ are the painful stiffening of a joint and muscle.

7. The nervous system is the ___control___ center and ___message___ center of the body.

8. The nervous system ___senses___ and interprets information from the environment outside the body.

9. Eyes, ears, tongue, nose, and skin relay impulses to ___nerves___.

10. The circulatory system is made up of the ___heart___, blood vessels, and ___blood___.

11. Blood carries food, ___oxygen___, and other needed substances to cells.

12. The circulatory system helps remove ___waste___ products from cells.

13. The ___lungs___ accomplish the process of respiration.

14. Two functions of the respiratory system involve bringing oxygen into the body and eliminating ___carbon dioxide___.

15. The urinary system eliminates waste products created by the cells through ___urine___.

16. The gastrointestinal system has two functions: ___digestion___ and ___elimination___.

17. The endocrine system is made up of glands that secrete
___hormones___.

18. Hormones regulate levels of
___sugar___
in the blood and
___calcium___
in the bones.

19. The function of the reproductive system is to allow human beings to
___reproduce___,
or create new human life.

20. Sex glands are called the
___gonads___.

21. The immune system fights
___infection___.

22. The lymphatic system removes excess
___fluids___ and
waste products from the body's tissues.

True or False.

Looking at the normal changes of aging for each body system, mark a "T" for true or an "F" for false.

23. _F_ A normal change of aging for the integumentary system is that skin gets more oily and becomes thicker.

24. _T_ An older person may feel colder because protective fatty tissue becomes thinner.

25. _T_ A person may lose height as she ages.

26. _F_ Bones become thicker and harder to break as a person ages.

27. _T_ A normal change of aging for the nervous system is slower responses and reflexes.

28. _F_ An older person will be extremely forgetful and unable to remember much of anything.

29. _T_ As a person ages, he may find it harder to taste or smell foods.

30. _T_ Narrowed blood vessels and decreased blood flow are normal changes of aging for the circulatory system.

31. _T_ The strength of the lungs decreases as a person ages.

32. _F_ The bladder holds more urine as a person ages, making urination less frequent.

33. _T_ A normal change of aging for the urinary system is that the bladder may not empty completely. This makes the risk higher for infection.

34. _T_ An older person may be constipated more frequently.

35. _F_ As a person ages, she may have a decrease of saliva and other digestive fluids.

36. _F_ An older person is more able to handle stress.

37. _T_ A decrease in progesterone and estrogen is a normal change of aging for the endocrine system.

38. _T_ For women, aging means a higher risk of osteoporosis due to a loss of calcium from a decrease in estrogen.

39. _F_ An older male will produce more sperm.

40. _T_ An older person will be at a higher risk for all types of infections.

41. _F_ A normal change of aging for the immune system is an increased response to vaccines.

Scenarios.

Read the following paragraphs and decide which items should be reported to the nurse.

Integumentary System

42. You are providing care for Mrs. Miller. As you are assisting her to turn over, you notice that she has a red spot above her buttocks and a bruise on her upper arm. Which items need to be reported to the nurse?

_____

_____

_____

_____

_____

Musculoskeletal System

43. You are providing care for Mr. Leary. As you assist him out of bed, he moves slowly. Today he is only able to walk a shorter distance than yesterday. He seems to be limping and occasionally makes a noise. Which items need to be reported to the nurse?

_____

_____

_____

_____

_____

Nervous System

44. You are assisting Ms. Rice with eating. It takes her a few seconds to take the napkin you are offering her. While she is eating, you notice she coughs while swallowing. She suddenly says that she cannot see the food on the left side of her plate. Which items need to be reported to the nurse?

_____

_____

_____

_____

_____

_____

Circulatory System

45. You are giving Mrs. Lee a bed bath. You notice that her fingertips are blue and her feet are swollen. She complains of being tired. Which items need to be reported to the nurse?

_____

_____

_____

_____

_____

Respiratory System

46. You are giving care to Mr. Martin. He makes a wheezing sound when he breathes out of his mouth. After turning him over, he says he needs to rest before continuing. He begins to cough. Which items need to be reported to the nurse?

_____

_____

_____

_____

Name: _____

Urinary System

47. You always need to give Mr. Parsons a urinal before and after you help him walk. Today you notice that his urine seems cloudy and foul-smelling. When you come in later, you find urine on his bed linens. Which items need to be reported to the nurse?

_____

_____

_____

_____

_____

_____

_____

Gastrointestinal System

48. Mr. Sanchez is not eating as much as he used to. He has lost two pounds since you last weighed him. He says he just isn't as hungry lately. Which items need to be reported to the nurse?

_____

_____

_____

_____

_____

_____

Endocrine System

49. You walk into Mrs. Walker's room and notice she has just finished drinking her water in the glass beside her bed. She asks you to refill her water pitcher because it's empty. You just filled it ten minutes ago. When you return with her pitcher, you see that she is sweating even

though she has no blanket over her and the room feels cool to you. Which items need to be reported to the nurse?

_____

_____

_____

_____

_____

_____

_____

Reproductive System

50. You offer Mr. Tadley a urinal because he requests it. He has trouble urinating and his face indicates that he is in pain. He later tells you he has a sore area on his penis. Which items need to be reported to the nurse?

_____

_____

_____

_____

_____

_____

_____

Lymphatic and Immune Systems

51. Ms. Gallagher is running a fever. She complains of being tired and mentions that she has had three bouts of diarrhea in the last hour. Which items need to be reported to the nurse?

_____

_____

_____

_____

Name: _____

Short Answer.

For each body system, write down two ways you can help your residents with their normal changes of aging. One example has been completed for you.

Integumentary System

1. Keep resident's skin clean and dry.

2. _____

   _____

   _____

Musculoskeletal System

1. _____

   _____

   _____

2. _____

   _____

   _____

Nervous System

1. _____

   _____

   _____

2. _____

   _____

   _____

Circulatory System

1. _____

   _____

   _____

2. _____

   _____

   _____

Respiratory System

1. _____

   _____

   _____

2. _____

   _____

   _____

Urinary System

1. _____

   _____

   _____

2. _____

   _____

   _____

Gastrointestinal System

1. _____

   _____

   _____

2. _____

   _____

   _____

Endocrine System

1. _____

   _____

   _____

2. _____

   _____

   _____

Reproductive System

1. _____

   _____

_____

2. _____

_____

_____

Lymphatic and Immune Systems

1. _____

_____

_____

2. _____

_____

_____

FIVE

Personal Care Skills

Unit 1: Explain personal care of residents

Fill in the Blank.

1. Skills you assist with and how much help you provide will depend on a resident's

   _____

   to do self-care.

2. Personal care is a very

   _____

   experience.

3. Be _____
   when assisting with personal care tasks.

4. Before you begin any task,

   _____

   to the resident exactly what you will be doing.

5. Ask if he or she would like to use the

   _____

   or bedpan first.

6. Personal care may be

   _____

   for some residents.

7. Provide the resident with

   _____.

8. During personal care,

   _____

   residents for any problems or changes that have occurred.

9. After care make sure the

   _____

   is within reach and the bed is left in its

   _____

   position.

10. If the resident appears tired, stop and take a short _____.

11. AM or PM care refers to the time of

    _____

    care tasks are performed.

Unit 2: Describe guidelines for assisting with bathing

True or False.

Mark each statement with either a "T" for true or "F" for false.

1. _____ Older skin produces less perspiration and oil.

2. _____ Check to make sure the bathroom or shower room floor is dry before bathing a resident.

3. _____ The face, hands, underarms, and perineum should be washed once a week.

4. _____ Checking the water temperature before bathing is not necessary.

5. _____ Bathing provides a great opportunity to observe a resident's skin.

6. _____ Have the resident use safety bars when getting into or out of the tub or shower.

7. _____ Checking to make sure the room is warm enough for the resident before bathing is important.

8. _____ Use bath oils when assisting a resident to take a tub bath.

Name: _____

9. _____ Covering a resident while transporting to and from shower or tub room provides warmth and privacy.

10. _____ Leave the resident alone while he or she is in the shower room.

Short Answer.

11. Think about your own routine for bathing. If you were unable to do it by yourself, how would you feel? Why is protecting a resident's privacy so important when bathing?

_____

_____

_____

_____

_____

_____

Unit 3: Describe guidelines for assisting with grooming

Multiple Choice.

Circle the letter of the answer that best completes the statement or answers the question.

1. Nail care should be provided:
   a. when a resident asks you to do it
   b. if it has specifically been assigned
   c. when you notice a resident's nails are getting long
   d. all of the above

2. Why should you never cut a resident's toenails, especially a diabetic resident's?
   a. Poor circulation can lead to infection if skin is accidentally cut.
   b. An infection can lead to a severe wound or even amputation.
   c. both a and b
   d. none of the above

3. How can you help promote independence and dignity while assisting with grooming?
   a. by allowing residents to do all they can for themselves
   b. by letting residents make as many choices as possible
   c. by following residents' personal routines or particular ways of grooming themselves
   d. all of the above

4. Briefly describe each razor.

A **safety** razor _____

_____

_____

_____

_____

_____

_____

An **electric** razor _____

_____

_____

_____

_____

_____

_____

A **disposable** razor_____

_____

_____

_____

_____

_____

_____

Unit 4: Identify guidelines for good oral hygiene

Crossword.

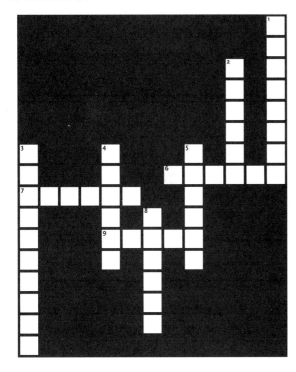

Clues:

Across

6. Canker sores or small, painful, white sores are examples of these, and they must be reported.

_____

7. Flossing the teeth removes tartar and this.

_____

9. How often oral care is performed, at least, per day

_____

Down

1. Artificial teeth

_____

2. Oral care needs to include brushing this too, along with the teeth

_____

3. The inhalation of food or drink into the lungs

_____

4. Breath that smells bad or like this must be reported.

_____

5. When providing oral care you must wear these in case the gums bleed.

_____

8. With unconscious residents, it is important to use this as little as possible when performing mouth care.

_____

Unit 5: List guidelines for assisting with dressing

Fill in the Blank.

1. If a resident has a weakened side from a stroke or injury, that side is called the _____ side.

2. Use the terms _____ or _____ to refer to the affected side.

3. The _____ arm is usually placed through a sleeve first.

4. Encourage a resident to dress in _____ clothes rather than nightclothes.

5. Encourage and allow a resident to _____ clothing for the day.

6. Place the weak arm or leg through the garment first, then the _____ arm.

7. Having residents choose the clothes they will wear encourages _____ and promotes self-care.

8. IV stands for

_____,

or into a vein.

9. Always keep an IV bag

_____

IV site on body.

10. Remove or assist in removing clothing from the side

_____

the IV first.

Unit 6: Explain guidelines for assisting with toileting

Matching.

Write the letter of the correct definition beside each term listed below.

a. A bedpan that is flatter than the regular bedpan.

b. Generally used by men for urination

c. A specific amount of water flowed into the colon to eliminate stool

d. An inability to control the muscles of the bowels or bladder

e. A chair with a toilet seat and a removable container underneath

f. A medication given rectally to cause a bowel movement

g. The inability to have a bowel movement

1. _____ constipation

2. _____ portable commode

3 _____ fracture pan

4. _____ enema

5. _____ urinal

6. _____ suppository

7. _____ incontinence

Labeling.

Identify the following elimination supplies.

8. _____
_____

9. _____
_____

10. _____
_____

Short Answer.

11. Why should you note the color, odor, and qualities of urine and stool after a resident uses a bedpan, urinal, or commode?

_____

_____

_____

_____

_____

_____

_____

_____

_____

_____

_____

Unit 7: Identify guidelines for good skin care

Labeling.

Label the pressure sore danger areas. Some areas have already been filled in for you.

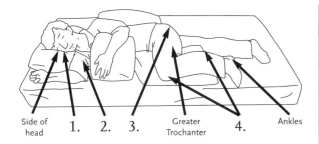

Side of head 1. 2. 3. Greater Trochanter 4. Ankles

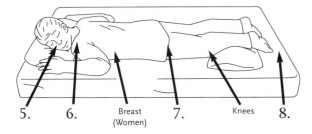

5. 6. Breast (Women) 7. Knees 8.

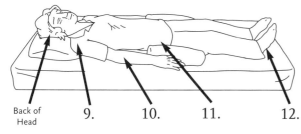

Back of Head 9. 10. 11. 12.

1. _____

2. _____

3. _____

4. _____

5. _____

6. _____

7. _____

8. _____

9. _____

10. _____

11. _____

12. _____

Multiple Choice.

Circle the letter of the answer that best completes the statement or answers the question.

13. Which of the following are conditions that increase the risk of pressure sores?

   a. warmth

   b. moisture

   c. pressure

   d. all of the above

14. Which of the following statements are true about pressure sores?

   a. Approximately 90% of pressure sores in nursing homes develop within the first three weeks of admission.

   b. Pressure sores are painful and difficult to heal. They can lead to life-threatening infection.

   c. Prevention of pressure sores is very important.

   d. all of the above

True or False.

Mark each statement with either a "T" for true or "F" for false.

15. _____ Rashes or any discoloration of the skin is something you should report.

16. _____ You should reposition residents who cannot get out of bed at least every two hours.

17. _____ Pull residents across the sheets during transfers or repositioning.

18. _____ Back rubs can help relax residents and increase their circulation.

19. _____ Residents seated in chairs or wheelchairs do not need to be repositioned.

20. _____ Sheepskin or bed pads absorb perspiration and protect the skin from irritating bed linens.

21. _____ Massage any white, red, or purple areas you see on a resident's skin.

Name: _____

Matching.

Write the letter of the correct definition beside each term listed below.

sheets placed under residents who are unable to assist with turning in bed, lifting, or moving up in bed

b. keep the fingers from curling tightly

c. used to keep the bed covers from pushing down on resident's feet.

d. padded boards placed against the resident's feet to keep them flexed

22. _____ bed cradles

23. _____ footboards

24. _____ hand rolls

25. _____ draw sheets

Unit 8: Explain the guidelines for safely transferring and positioning residents

Multiple Choice.

Circle the letter of the answer that best completes the statement or answers the question.

1. To minimize the manual lifting of residents, you should:
    a. use the provided equipment properly
    b. work by yourself to transfer or reposition a resident
    c. bend at the waist while lifting
    d. none of the above

2. When a resident falls:
    a. widen your stance and bring the resident's body close to you
    b. catch the resident under the arms to stop the fall
    c. try to reverse the fall
    d. all of the above

3. All of the following statements are true about wheelchairs, except:

a. The wheelchair should be unlocked before assisting a resident into or out of it.

b. You should know how to apply and release the brake and how to operate the footrests.

c. After a transfer, a wheelchair should be unlocked.

d. Ask the resident how you can assist with wheelchairs. Some residents will want you to be more involved with the transfer.

4. A sliding or transfer board:
    a. may be used to help transfer residents who are unable to bear weight on their legs
    b. can be used for almost any transfer that involves moving from one sitting position to another
    c. fits around the resident's waist outside her clothing
    d. both a and b

5. When putting a transfer belt on a resident, leave enough room to:
    a. insert the resident's knees into the belt
    b. insert your shoulder into the belt
    c. insert two fingers into the belt
    d. none of the above

Short Answer.

6. Why is it important to understand and use provided equipment when lifting or transferring a resident?

_____
_____
_____
_____
_____

SIX

Basic Nursing Skills

Unit 1: Explain admission, transfer, and discharge of a resident

Word Search.

Complete each of the following sentences and find your answers in the word search.

```
r l q s n o i t s e u q r k
u j l t u t y y m x e u m g
m v r x i m f d w a s w a d
j f f x s m q o r h y o g m
e u l l r h p e r w z c g s
v k q j o t f r t m d d i v
c o c n k u p m e s a n j o
i n i n l r o n e s u l j y
h o p l e e s j p a s j x e
g f y p g b s j j d q i d f
m z a n h o l t k h w o a
x r a x n w e l q u g e c n
e h p o s i t i v e d d e d
c h e k x e c u d o r t n i
```

1. Moving into a nursing home is a big *change* .

2. Make sure a resident has a good *impression* of you and your facility.

3. Answer any *questions* a new resident has.

4. Never *rush* the process or the new resident.

5. Handle personal possessions *carefully* and respectfully.

6. *Introduce* the resident to all staff members and residents you see.

7. *Prepare* the room before the resident arrives.

8. Always address the person with his *last formal* name until he tells you how he wants to be addressed.

9. To lessen the stress of a transfer, inform the resident as soon as possible so he can begin to *adjust* to the idea.

10. For a resident who is being discharged, be *positive* . Assure the resident he is ready for this important change.

Short Answer.

11. Why do you think it's important to make a new resident feel comfortable?

_____
_____
_____
_____
_____
_____
_____

Name: _____

Unit 2: Explain the importance of monitoring vital signs

Short Answer.

The four sites for taking body temperature are:

1. _____

   _____

2. _____

   _____

3. _____

   _____

4. _____

   _____

Watching for changes in vital signs is important. What changes in vital signs need to be reported to the nurse right away?

5. _____

   _____

   _____

6. _____

   _____

   _____

7. _____

   _____

   _____

8. _____

   _____

   _____

List the normal ranges for vital signs.

Temperature: Fahrenheit   Celsius

9. Oral_____

10. Rectal _____

11. Axillary _____

12. Pulse_____

13. Respirations_____

   _____

14. Blood Pressure_____

   _____

15. Why do you need to handle a mercury thermometer with care?

   _____

   _____

   _____

   _____

   _____

   _____

16. Why should you record vital signs immediately?

   _____

   _____

   _____

   _____

   _____

17. Why should you count respirations immediately after taking the pulse?

   _____

   _____

   _____

   _____

   _____

   _____

   _____

Matching.

Write the letter of the correct definition beside each term listed below.

a. brachial pulse

b. respiration

c. radial pulse

d. inspiration

e. diastolic

f. expiration

g. systolic

18. _____ A measurement of blood pressure showing when the heart is at work, contracting and pushing blood out of the left ventricle

19. _____ The process of breathing air into the lungs and exhaling air out of the lungs

20. _____ The most common site for checking the pulse, located on the inside of the wrist, where the radial artery runs just beneath the skin

21. _____ A measurement of blood pressure showing when the heart relaxes

22. _____ The pulse inside the elbow, about 1–1½ inches above the elbow

23. _____ Breathing air into the lungs

24. _____ Exhaling air out of the lungs

Labeling.

Label the four main types of thermometers.

25. _____

26. _____

27. _____

28. _____

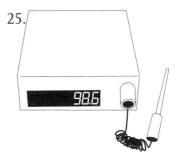

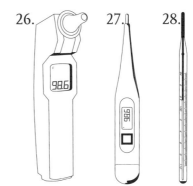

Unit 3: Explain how to measure height and weight

True or False.

Mark each statement with either a "T" for true or "F" for false.

1. _____ If a resident loses one pound, you do not need to report it.

2. _____ On some wheelchair scales, you will need to subtract the weight of the wheelchair before recording a resident's weight.

3. _____ If a resident is unable to get out of bed, a special scale can be used to weigh him or her.

4. _____ Residents who are unable to get out of bed cannot have their height measured.

5. _____ For a resident who is bed-bound, you will have to measure height by making marks on the sheet with a pencil at the top of the resident's head and at the bottom of the feet.

6. _____ You can measure the height of a resident who has contractures.

Name: _____

Labeling.

Looking at the scale below, how much does this resident weigh?

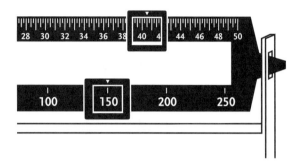

7._____

Unit 4: Explain restraints and how to promote a restraint-free environment

Multiple Choice.

Circle the letter of the answer that best completes the statement or answers the question.

1. A restraint is a physical or chemical way to limit a person's movement. An example of restraining a resident includes:

    a. tying his legs and arms to the bed

    b. putting both side rails up on the bed

    c. giving him medication to calm him down

    d. all of the above

2. A serious problem that has been associated with restraints includes:

    a. pressure sores

    b. death

    c. both a and b

    d. none of the above

3. Restraints can be applied:

    a. as punishment from staff when a resident isn't behaving properly

    b. only with a doctor's order

    c. when a staff member doesn't have time to watch a resident closely

    d. none of the above

4. An example of a restraint alternative is:

    a. Assisting a resident to the bathroom

    b. Giving a resident a repetitive task

    c. Answering a call light promptly

    d. all of the above

Short Answer.

5. When a resident is restrained, he or she has to be monitored continuously. The resident must be checked at least every 30 minutes. What needs to happen every two hours, or as needed?

    _____

    _____

    _____

    _____

    _____

    _____

    _____

    _____

    _____

    _____

6. How do you think you would feel if you were restrained? Can you understand why it might make someone feel a loss of dignity or feel depressed?

    _____

    _____

    _____

    _____

Unit 5: Define fluid balance and explain intake and output (I&O)

Fill in the Blank.

1. _____

    is maintaining the intake and output of fluids.

2. Fluid balance requires taking in the

   _____

   amount of fluid as the body puts out.

3. A _____
   is a tube used to drain urine from the
   bladder.

4. A catheter drainage bag must always be
   kept _____
   than the hips or bladder.

5. Catheter tubing should be kept as

   _____

   as possible and should not be

   _____.

6. An indwelling catheter remains inside
   the _____
   for a period of time.

7. _____ and
   _____ are
   two types of specimens you may be
   asked to collect from a resident.

8. _____
   is mucus coughed up from the lungs.

9. A _____
   urine specimen does not include the
   first and last urine in the sample.

10. When cleaning catheter tubing, clean at
    least _____
    inches of it nearest meatus. Move in
    only one direction,

    _____

    from meatus. Use a

    _____

    area of the cloth for each stroke.

Short Answer.

11. How many cubic centimeters (cc) equal
    1 ounce (oz.)?

    _____

    _____

    _____

Unit 6: Explain care guidelines for different types of tubing

Mark an X by all of the correct guidelines for working with residents who have gastric tubes.

1. _____ Make sure that tubing is kinked.

2. _____ Only doctors or nurses insert or remove tubes.

3. _____ During the feeding, the resident should remain in a sitting position with the head of the bed elevated about 45 degrees.

4. _____ Provide frequent mouth care.

5. _____ Keep resident on top of the tubing.

6. _____ Nursing assistants perform tube feedings.

7. _____ Watch for signs of infection, including redness or drainage around the opening.

Mark an X by all of the correct guidelines for working around oxygen equipment.

8. _____ Smoking is okay in the room or area where oxygen is used or stored.

9. _____ Remove all fire hazards from the room or area.

10. _____ Fire hazards can be electric shavers, hair dryers, or other electrical appliances.

11. _____ Nursing assistants can adjust oxygen levels.

12. _____ Never allow candles or other open flames around oxygen.

13. _____ Check behind the ears for irritation from nasal cannula.

Name: _____

Short Answer.

14. List eight items to report about an IV.

_____

_____

_____

_____

_____

_____

_____

_____

_____

_____

_____

_____

Unit 7: Explain the importance of sleep and perform proper bedmaking

Crossword.

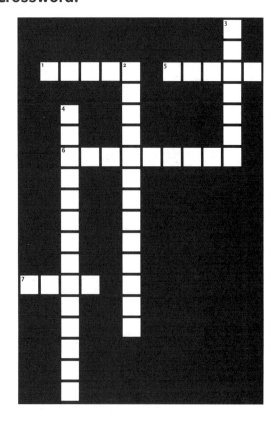

Clues:

Across

1. Provides the body with new cells and energy

   _____

5. You don't bend at the waist to make a bed. You bend these.

   _____

6. A bed completely made with the bedspread and blankets in place

   _____

7. You carry linen this way when collecting it to make a bed—

   _____

   from your uniform.

Down

2. Residents who spend long hours in bed are at risk for these.

   _____

3. Turn a closed bed into this by folding the linen down to the foot of the bed.

   _____

4. These thrive in moist, warm environments.

   _____

Unit 8: Explain how to apply non-sterile dressings

Fill in the Blank.

1. Sterile dressings are those that cover _____ or _____ wounds. A _____ always changes these dressings. Non-sterile dressings are applied to_____ wounds that have less chance of

   _____.

SEVEN

Nutrition and Hydration

Unit 1: Identify the six basic nutrients and the USDA Food Guide Pyramid

Read the following sentences and mark which of the six basic nutrients it is describing. Use a "P" for proteins, "C" for carbohydrates, "F" for fats, "V" for vitamins, "M" for minerals, and "W" for water.

1. _____ Good sources of these are fish, meat, dried beans, and cheese.

2. _____ Without this, a person can only live a few days.

3. _____ These help the body store energy.

4. _____ It protects organs and helps the body absorb certain vitamins.

5. _____ Beans and rice are examples of complementary _____.

6. _____ Examples of these are butter, oil, and salad dressing.

7. _____ They are essential for tissue growth and repair.

8. _____ Most of these cannot be produced by the body.

9. _____ Simple _____ are stored as fat.

10. _____ Examples of these include bread, cereal, and potatoes.

11. _____ This is the most essential nutrient for life.

12. _____ Through perspiration, this helps to maintain body temperature.

13. _____ These can be fat-soluble or water-soluble.

14. _____ One-half to two-thirds of our body weight is this.

15. _____ Iron and calcium are examples of these.

Labeling.

Looking at the Food Guide Pyramid below, fill in the six food groups.

16. _____

17. _____

18. _____

19. _____

20. _____

21. _____

Name: _____

_____

_____

_____

_____

_____

Read the following descriptions and mark which of the six food groups they are describing—"G" for grains, "FR" for fruits, "V" for vegetables, "D" for dairy products, "M" for meat, poultry, etc., "F" for fats.

22. _____ One of the best sources of vitamin C; one serving from this group could include one medium-sized apple, orange, or banana.

23. _____ These foods provide protein, minerals, and vitamins. In addition, some are a good source of iron.

24. _____ Excellent sources of vitamins and fiber; lettuce, spinach, kale; tomatoes, green beans, and broccoli are examples.

25. _____ These provide calcium for healthy bones and teeth. One serving from this group could include one cup of milk or yogurt, one-half cup of cottage cheese, or one-and-a-half ounces of cheese.

26. _____ These are found in cereal, bread, rice, and pasta. They are a great source of carbohydrates.

27. _____ These contain more than twice as many calories per gram as carbohydrates or proteins. They should be eaten in small quantities.

Unit 2: Demonstrate an awareness of regional, cultural, and religious food preferences

Short Answer.

1. Briefly describe some of the foods you ate while growing up. Were there any special dishes that your family made that were related to your culture, religion, or region?

_____

Unit 3: Explain special diets

Matching.

Read the following sentences and identify what special diet it is describing. Choose from the diets listed below.

a. Low-Sodium Diet

b. Fluid-Restricted Diet

c. Low-Protein Diet

d. Low-Fat/Low-Cholesterol Diet

e. Modified Calorie Diet

f. Dietary Management of Ulcers

g. Dietary Management of Diabetes

1. _____ To prevent further heart or kidney damage, physicians may restrict a resident's fluid intake.

2. _____ In addition to restricted intake of fluids and sodium, people who have kidney disease may also be on this diet.

3. _____ People at risk for heart attacks and heart disease may be placed on these. This diet includes limiting fatty meats, egg yolks, and fried foods.

4. _____ Calories and carbohydrates must be carefully regulated in this diet. The types of foods and the amounts are determined by the person's nutritional and energy requirements.

5. _____ Salt is restricted in this diet. Other high sodium foods, such as ham,

nuts, pickles, and canned soups, will be limited.

6. _____ Used for losing weight or preventing additional weight gain.

7. _____ This diet avoids foods that increase the levels of acid in the stomach. Alcohol, beverages containing caffeine, and spicy seasonings are some of the things that should be avoided.

Unit 4: Understand the importance of observing and reporting a resident's diet

Short Answer.

1. What are two common food errors for residents on special diets?

_____

_____

_____

_____

_____

_____

_____

_____

2. What are two reasons you should observe what a resident eats?

_____

_____

_____

_____

_____

_____

_____

_____

Unit 5: Describe how to assist residents in maintaining fluid balance

Fill in the Blank.

1. The sense of _____ can lessen as people age.

2. Most residents should be encouraged to drink _____ to _____ glasses of water a day.

3. _____ occurs when a person does not have enough fluid in the body.

4. Encourage residents to

_____

every time you see them.

5. Offer fresh _____ or other fluids often.

6. Make sure pitcher and cup are near enough and _____ enough for the resident to lift.

7. If appropriate, offer sips of liquid

_____

bites of food at meals and snacks.

8. _____ occurs when the body is unable to handle the amount of fluid consumed.

Short Answer.

9. List ten things to observe and report about dehydration.

_____

_____

_____

_____

_____

_____

_____

_____

Name: _____

_____
_____
_____
_____
_____
_____
_____
_____

e	u	a	x	w	e	r	a	c	l	a	r	o	u
e	k	j	i	l	n	s	t	u	m	b	b	p	s
j	e	a	e	j	e	t	s	w	y	e	r	y	e
l	r	t	t	p	s	f	l	v	v	i	g	z	c
q	c	x	i	n	z	k	n	e	g	p	a	p	d
l	j	o	f	t	i	g	r	h	p	y	e	p	o
i	v	p	i	c	e	a	t	u	e	s	v	b	h
b	w	m	v	m	g	p	c	m	d	v	a	a	x
j	n	o	u	e	j	z	p	l	u	j	q	l	m
d	o	q	s	w	f	z	l	a	o	b	w	m	w
t	a	t	d	b	n	t	o	x	m	e	c	l	p
c	a	o	o	u	d	x	g	e	k	d	m	z	n
e	o	w	i	x	v	a	g	c	c	d	c	i	u
f	u	t	e	n	s	i	l	s	i	i	w	c	t

10. List six things to observe and report about fluid overload.

_____
_____ .
_____
_____
_____
_____
_____
_____
_____
_____
_____
_____
_____
_____
_____
_____
_____

1. Encourage residents to
   _____.

2. Provide _____
   before and after meals.

3. Honor _____
   likes and dislikes.

4. Offer many different kinds of foods and
   _____.

5. Allow enough _____
   to finish eating.

6. Notify nurse if resident has trouble
   using _____.

7. Position residents sitting
   _____ for feeding.

8. If resident has had a loss of
   _____,
   ask about it.

9. Record meal/snack
   _____.

Unit 6: List ways to identify and prevent unintended weight loss

Word Search.

Complete each of the following sentences and find your answers in the word search.

Unit 7: Identify ways to promote appetites at mealtime

Short Answer.

Read the following paragraph and answer the question.

Susana, a nursing assistant, enters Mr. Franti's room to assist him with his dinner. She tells him hello and asks him if he would like to wear a clothing protector while dining. He says yes. She applies the protector and brings the tray over. She cuts his food into small pieces and notices that his meat is almost cold. She offers him a fork. He can't grasp it so she begins feeding him herself. She stares out the window while offering him bites. He says that he is finished. She looks down and notices that he has barely touched his food.

1. What are some ways that Susana could have better promoted her resident's appetite? What important things did she forget? What did she do right?

_____
_____
_____
_____
_____
_____
_____
_____
_____
_____
_____
_____
_____
_____
_____
_____
_____
_____
_____

Unit 8: Demonstrate ways to feed residents

Multiple Choice.

Circle the correct response.

1. When assisting residents with eating, encourage them to do whatever they can for themselves. This includes:

    a. if a resident can hold a napkin, she should

    b. if a resident can use special adaptive utensils, she should

    c. if a resident can hold and eat finger foods, she should

    d. all of the above

2. Ways to promote a resident's dignity while feeding include:

    a. Telling him, "Hurry up. I've got three other people to feed."

    b. Asking him, "What would you like to try first?"

    c. Looking around the room while he is eating

    d. none of the above

True or False.

Mark each statement with either a "T" for true or "F" for false.

3. _____ If a resident says, "I don't want to wear a clothing protector," you should put one on her anyway.

4. _____ Residents who must be fed are often embarrassed and depressed about their dependence on another person.

5. _____ Alternate food and drink while feeding.

6. _____ Sit higher than a resident while feeding.

Name: _____

7. _____ You should give a resident your full attention during eating.

8. _____ When feeding a resident, make sure the resident's mouth is empty before giving another bite of food or sip of beverage.

9. _____ A resident should be fed lying flat on his back.

Unit 9: Describe eating and swallowing problems a resident may have

Short Answer.

1. List five ways to prevent aspiration.

_____

_____

_____

_____

_____

_____

_____

_____

_____

_____

_____

_____

_____

_____

_____

_____

Fill in the Blank.

2. A _____ tube is inserted into the nose going to the stomach. A

_____ tube is inserted through the abdomen, into the stomach. With

_____

_____ a resident receives nutrients directly into the bloodstream.

EIGHT

Common, Chronic, and Acute Conditions

Unit 1: Describe common diseases and disorders of the musculoskeletal system

Short Answer.

Look at the guidelines for caring for a resident with arthritis. Answer the following questions.

1. Mr. Garcia, a resident with arthritis, says his stomach hurts. What should you do?

   _____

   _____

   _____

   _____

   _____

   _____

   _____

2. Mrs. Johnson, a resident with arthritis, doesn't want to go on a walk. She has refused to walk the last few times you've gone into her room. What can you do?

   _____

   _____

   _____

   _____

   _____

   _____

   _____

3. Mr. Knight, a resident with arthritis, has

always dressed himself. Lately, he has had a hard time pulling on his pants and socks. What can you do?

   _____

   _____

   _____

   _____

   _____

   _____

   _____

   _____

   _____

Fill in the Blank.

4. Brittle bones mean that the bones can _____ easily.

5. _____,

   _____,

   and _____
   are used to treat osteoporosis.

6. Nursing assistants must

   _____

   and _____
   residents with osteoporosis very carefully.

7. A broken bone is called a

   _____.

8. Preventing _____, which can lead to fractures, is very important.

9. After hip replacement surgery, a person is not able to _____ on that leg while the hip heals.

Name: _____

Word Search.

Look at the guidelines and observing and reporting for hip replacement. Complete each of the following sentences and find your answers in the word search.

e	r	u	s	h	u	n	m	m	n	f	a	v	n
t	n	o	t	z	l	w	x	n	u	v	t	e	c
g	q	e	e	i	x	c	h	p	u	g	u	z	f
v	e	c	r	p	d	q	b	m	h	x	f	v	h
k	t	i	c	g	e	k	m	t	x	e	x	c	d
k	z	x	e	w	y	b	b	j	t	x	a	e	a
a	a	h	i	v	v	q	k	i	v	e	t	w	q
f	x	s	a	y	c	s	c	q	r	c	w	q	j
d	q	i	n	b	r	i	g	r	e	t	g	o	t
g	g	d	j	a	k	d	z	f	o	k	f	l	c
s	t	p	e	m	p	n	f	r	z	s	d	z	k
s	i	z	b	a	c	a	r	f	p	y	s	s	r
h	a	c	o	t	k	q	y	e	c	z	o	e	f
y	u	z	m	t	y	q	n	d	n	e	o	s	d

10. Keep often-used items within

   _____ .

11. Dress starting with the

   _____

   side first.

12. Never _____
   the resident. Use praise and encouragement.

13. Have the resident sit to do tasks and
   save _____ .

14. Caution the resident not to sit with legs
   _____ .

Report these signs to the nurse:

15. if incision is _____ ,
   draining, or _____
   to touch

16. an increase in _____

17. abnormal _____ ,
   especially elevated temperature

18. following doctor's orders for activity and

   _____

Short Answer.

Looking at the two illustrations below, which one is showing a 90 degree angle? A person recovering form hip replacement cannot bend the hip at an angle less than this.

a.   b.

19. _____

   _____

   _____

   _____

   _____

Unit 2: Describe common diseases and disorders of the nervous system

Looking at the care guidelines for residents with Alzheimer's, for each of the following statements write "yes" if the statement is correct, and "no" if the statement is incorrect.

1. _____ Use nonslip mats, tub seats, and hand holds to ensure safety during bathing.

2. _____ Always bathe the resident at the same time every day, even if he or she is agitated.

3. _____ Always use the same steps and explain what you are doing the same way every time.

4. _____ Do not attempt to groom the resident, since he or she may not enjoy this.

5. _____ Mark the restroom with a sign as a reminder of when to use it and where it is.

6. _____ Do not encourage exercise as this will make the resident more agitated.

7. _____ Do not encourage independence as this can lead to aggressive behavior.

8. _____ Share in enjoyable activities.

9. _____ Reward positive behavior with smiles, hugs, warm touches, and thank yous.

Short Answer.

Choose which creative therapy for Alzheimer's disease is being described in each sentence.

Activity Therapy
Reality Orientation
Reminiscence Therapy
Validation Therapy

10. Encouraging the resident to talk about the past and explore memories.

_____

11. Using calendars, clocks, signs, and lists to help the resident remember who and where she is.

_____

12. Using activities to prevent boredom and frustration and improve self-esteem.

_____

13. Letting the resident believe he lives in the past or in imaginary circumstances, without attempting to reorient him.

_____

14. Encouraging residents to remember and talk about the past. Exploring memories by asking about details.

_____

Short Answer.

For each of the following personal attitudes in caring for Alzheimer's residents, briefly describe why the attitude is helpful.

15. Don't take their behavior personally. Why?

_____
_____
_____
_____
_____
_____
_____
_____
_____

16. Put yourself in their shoes. Why?

_____
_____
_____
_____
_____
_____
_____
_____

17. Work with the symptoms and behaviors you see. Why?

_____
_____
_____
_____
_____
_____
_____
_____

18. Work as a team. Why?

_____

_____

_____

_____

_____

_____

_____

19. Take care of yourself. Why?

_____

_____

_____

_____

_____

_____

_____

_____

20. Work with family members. Why?

_____

_____

_____

_____

_____

_____

_____

21. Remember the goals of the resident care plan. Why?

_____

_____

_____

_____

_____

_____

_____

_____

True or False.

Mark each statement with either a "T" for true or "F" for false.

22. _____ When communicating with an Alzheimer's resident, speak in a calm, quiet manner.

23. _____ Plenty of noise and distractions can help the resident cope with having Alzheimer's disease.

24. _____ Perseveration means to wander constantly.

25. _____ When working with an Alzheimer's resident, you may have to repeat yourself several times.

26. _____ You should always use the same words and phrases when repeating something.

27. _____ Parkinson's disease causes stooped posture and a shuffling gait, or walk.

28. _____ A drawing of a toilet can be a form of communication.

29. _____ Restlessness, hunger, need for toileting, and pain may cause pacing and wandering.

30. _____ If a resident with Alzheimer's hits you, it is okay to hit him back.

31. _____ Distracting a resident with AD with a simple, calm activity can help with sundowning.

32. _____ Dementia is a normal part of aging.

33. _____ Alzheimer's disease can be cured.

34. _____ Symptoms of Multiple Sclerosis include blurred vision, tremors, poor balance, and difficulty walking.

35. _____ Each person with AD will show different symptoms at different times.

36. _____ Encouraging residents with AD to perform ADLs and keep their minds and bodies as active as possible is important.

Scenarios.

Read each of the following statements, and answer the questions.

Kate, a nursing assistant, is getting ready to take Mr. Elliot, who is recovering from a stroke, on a walk. Mr. Elliot has difficulty communicating and suffers from confusion. "Let's see," Jody says. "We can walk to the gardens, the activity room, or the front area. Now, where would you like to go?"

37. What is wrong with the way Kate is communicating with Mr. Elliot?

_____

_____

_____

_____

_____

_____

_____

Kate notices that Mr. Elliot seems to be having trouble saying words clearly. He is

beginning to get frustrated because he can't tell Kate what he wants. Kate decides to ask only yes or no questions, so she tells Mr. Elliot, "If you find it too difficult to speak right now, why don't you try nodding your head for 'yes' and shaking your head for 'no'."

38. What is Kate doing right?

_____

_____

_____

_____

_____

_____

_____

_____

_____

_____

Fill in the Blank.

39. When assisting with a transfer for a resident with one-sided weakness, always lead with the _____ side.

40. Dress the _____ side first. This prevents unnecessary

_____ and _____ of the limb.

41. Undress the

_____ side first.

42. _____ is used to help the resident dress himself.

43. When assisting a resident to eat, be sure to place the food in the resident's

_____.

Name: _____

True or False.

Mark each statement with either a "T" for true or "F" for false.

44. _____ Residents with paralysis or loss of movement do not need physical therapy.

45. _____ Leg exercises improve circulation.

46. _____ When assisting with eating, make sure food has been swallowed before offering more.

47. _____ When helping with transfers or ambulation, stand on the resident's stronger side.

48. _____ Always use a gait belt for safety.

49. _____ Refer to the side that has been affected by stroke as the "weaker" or "involved" side.

50. _____ Gestures and facial expressions are important in communicating with a resident who has had a stroke.

51. _____ Residents who suffer confusion or memory loss due to a stroke may feel more secure if you establish a routine of care.

52. _____ Residents may cry for no reason after suffering a stroke.

53. _____ When assisting a resident with eating, place food in the weaker or affected side of the mouth.

54. _____ Let the resident do things for him or herself whenever possible.

55. _____ "Yes" or "no" questions are best to use with a resident who has had a stroke.

56. _____ Dress the stronger side first when assisting with dressing.

Short Answer.

57. Which illustration shows a proper transfer of a resident with a one-sided weakness?

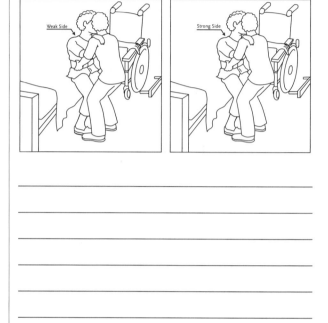

_____

_____

_____

_____

_____

_____

Unit 3: Describe common diseases and disorders of the circulatory system

Crossword.

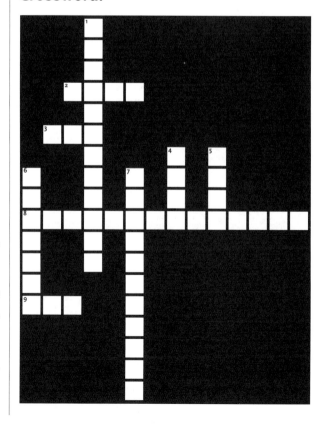

Clues:

Across

2. Some people complain of pain radiating down the inside of this arm.

_____

3. Residents may be on a diet that is low in this after suffering a heart attack.

_____

8. The condition that occurs when blood flow to the heart muscle is completely blocked and the muscle cell dies

_____

9. The abbreviation for the condition of blood backing up into the heart instead of circulating

_____

Down

1. Another name for high blood pressure

_____

4. PVD causes legs, feet, arms or hands to not have enough blood circulation. Skin may be this color.

_____

5. With angina pectoris, this is extremely important. It reduces the heart's need for extra oxygen. It helps the blood flow return to normal, often within three to fifteen minutes.

_____

6. These kind of leg stockings may be applied to reduce swelling in feet and ankles.

_____

7. Another name for chest pain

_____

Unit 4: Describe common diseases and disorders of the respiratory system

Multiple Choice.

Circle the letter of the answer that best completes the statement.

1. An infection of the lungs usually treated with antibiotics to reduce congestion and inflammation is:
   a. heart attack
   b. pneumonia
   c. urinary tract infection
   d. high blood pressure

2. Residents with COPD have difficulty with this:
   a. breathing
   b. urination
   c. weight
   d. vision

3. A constant fear of a person who has COPD is:
   a. constipation
   b. incontinence
   c. not being able to breathe
   d. heart attack

4. Residents who have COPD can experience the following:
   a. poor appetites
   b. lack of sleep
   c. fear of suffocation
   d. all of the above

5. A resident with COPD should be positioned:
   a. lying flat on his back
   b. sitting upright
   c. lying on his stomach
   d. lying on his side

6. Your role in caring for a resident with COPD includes:

   a. being calm and supportive

   b. encouraging independence with ADLs

   c. practicing good infection control

   d. all of the above

Short Answer.

7. Which illustration shows a more comfortable position for residents with COPD

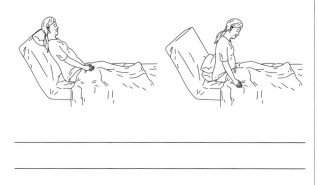

_____

_____

_____

_____

Unit 5: Describe common diseases and disorders of the urinary system

Fill in the Blank.

1. Females should always wipe from _____ to _____ after elimination.

2. UTIs are more common in _____.

3. UTIs result in a painful _____ feeling during urination. They also cause a frequent feeling of needing to _____.

4. Encourage _____.

5. Offer bedpan or a trip to the toilet at least every _____ hours. Answer call lights promptly.

6. Report _____ urine or if a resident urinates

   _____

   and in small quantities to the nurse.

Unit 6: Describe common diseases and disorders of the gastrointestinal system

Multiple Choice.

Circle the letter of the answer that best completes the statement.

1. The surgical removal of a portion of the intestines is called:

   a. an ostomy

   b. a nasogastric tube

   c. tracheostomy

   d. none of the above

2. Many residents with ostomies feel they have lost control of a basic bodily function. They may be embarrassed or angry about the ostomy. You should:

   a. be sensitive

   b. be supportive

   c. provide privacy

   d. all of the above

3. How often should an ostomy bag be emptied?

   a. whenever a stool is eliminated

   b. every ten minutes

   c. every 30 minutes

   d. when it's clean

4. Residents with ostomies should receive good skin care because:

   a. stool is irritating to the skin

   b. the ostomy bag is attached to the skin by adhesive

   c. both a and b

   d. none of the above

Unit 7: Describe common diseases and disorders of the endocrine system

Short Answer.

1. List six symptoms that people with diabetes may have.

_____

_____

_____

_____

_____

_____

_____

_____

_____

2. Why must diabetics be very careful about what they eat? How can diabetics make it easier to track what they should eat?

_____

_____

_____

_____

_____

_____

_____

_____

3. Why must nursing assistants only perform foot care for diabetics as directed?

_____

_____

_____

_____

_____

_____

_____

_____

4. List three important things nursing assistants can do when caring for residents with diabetes.

_____

_____

_____

_____

_____

_____

_____

_____

_____

_____

_____

_____

_____

_____

_____

Unit 8: Describe common diseases and disorders of the reproductive system

Fill in the Blank.

1. Older men often develop problems with the _____
gland. Prostate problems can include enlargement or, sometimes,

_____.

Either causes difficulty

_____

and/or _____
the bladder. _____
may be performed for cancer or to make the person more comfortable with elimination. Inform the nurse if you notice a
_____ urine stream or a lack of urination.

Name: _____

Unit 9: Describe common diseases and disorders of the lymphatic and immune systems

Multiple Choice.

Circle the letter of the answer that best completes the statement.

1. Care for the person with AIDS should focus on:
   a. helping to find a cure for HIV
   b. preventing transmission of HIV to others
   c. providing relief of symptoms and preventing complications
   d. none of the above

2. HIV is spread through:
   a. sex
   b. blood
   c. infected needles
   d. none of the above

3. AIDS residents who have infections of the mouth may need to eat food that is:
   a. spicy
   b. low in acid
   c. dry
   d. none of the above

4. Painful lesions in the mouth may be relieved by:
   a. drinking orange juice
   b. brushing them with a toothbrush
   c. rinsing frequently with warm salt water
   d. none of the above

5. Someone who has nausea and vomiting should:
   a. eat small frequent meals
   b. avoid high-fat and spicy foods
   c. drink liquids and eat salty foods
   d. none of the above

6. The "BRAT" diet is helpful for:
   a. diarrhea
   b. weight gain
   c. nausea and vomiting
   d. none of the above

7. People with AIDS often suffer from anxiety and depression because:
   a. AIDS cannot be cured.
   b. Others may have negative attitudes about people with AIDS.
   c. They have already lost friends and family members to the disease.
   d. all of the above

Mark the American Cancer Society's seven warning signs of cancer below.

8. _____ Change in bowel or bladder habits

9. _____ Difficulty breathing

10. _____ Dizziness

11. _____ Thickening or lump in breast

12. _____ Memory loss

13. _____ Obvious change in wart or mole

14. _____ Pain or swelling of the joints

15. _____ Persistent hoarseness or nagging cough

16. _____ Persistent indigestion or difficulty swallowing

17. _____ Nausea or vomiting

18. _____ Sweet, fruity breath odor

19. _____ Sore that does not heal

20. _____ Unusual bleeding or discharge from body opening

21. _____ Headache

Short Answer.

Briefly describe what your role is in caring for the resident with cancer with the items listed.

22. Communication

_____

_____

_____

_____

_____

23. Nutrition

_____

_____

_____

_____

_____

24. Pain control

_____

_____

_____

_____

_____

25. Skin care

_____

_____

_____

_____

_____

26. Oral care

_____

_____

_____

_____

27. Odor control

_____

_____

_____

_____

_____

28. Self-image

_____

_____

_____

_____

_____

29. Psychosocial needs

_____

_____

_____

_____

_____

30. Family assistance

_____

_____

_____

_____

_____

Unit 10: Describe mental illness, depression and related care

Scenarios.

Read each of the following scenarios, putting yourself in the resident's position, and then answer the questions for each scenario.

Annie, a nursing assistant, is taking care of a resident who is depressed. Annie is worried about Mrs. Rogers. She hurriedly dresses Mrs. Rogers even though Mrs. Rogers usually dresses herself. Annie says, "We don't want you to start crying today like you did yesterday."

1. What is Annie doing wrong?

_____

_____

_____

_____

_____

_____

_____

_____

Bruce, a nursing assistant, is taking care of a mentally ill resident who is verbally aggressive. The resident will sometimes yell at Bruce and accuse him of things. One day as Bruce is helping the resident eat, the resident starts yelling: "I hate spaghetti. You always make me eat it, and it makes my stomach hurt. You want me to be sick! Just leave me alone!"

2. Which of the following is the best response that Bruce can make?

a. "You have to eat this spaghetti because it's good for you."

b. "I'm sorry, I didn't realize you didn't like it. Would you like something else to eat instead?"

c. "You always say things like that. Of course you don't mean any of it. Just eat it, okay?"

d. If you don't eat this, you won't get any dessert."

NINE

Rehabilitation and Restorative Services

Unit 1: Describe the nursing assistant's role in rehabilitation

Short Answer.

1. What is rehabilitation?

_____

_____

_____

_____

_____

_____

2. What are restorative services?

_____

_____

_____

_____

_____

_____

3. What are three important things that you should do during rehabilitation?

_____

_____

_____

_____

_____

_____

Unit 2: List ways to promote a resident's independence

Short Answer.

1. Why is it important for a resident to remain as independent as possible?

_____

_____

_____

_____

_____

_____

2. List five things that a lack of mobility may result in.

_____

_____

_____

_____

_____

3. What six factors do regular ambulation and exercise help improve?

_____

_____

62

Name: _____

_____
_____
_____
_____
_____
_____

Unit 3: Describe assistive devices and equipment

Crossword.

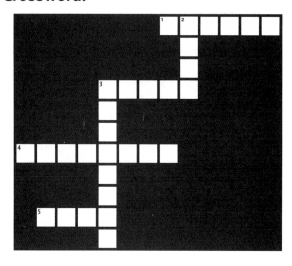

Clues:

Across

1. It is used when the resident can bear some weight on the legs. It provides stability for residents who are unsteady or lack balance.

_____

3. Examples of personal care adaptive equipment are long-handled brushes and _____.

4. Type of devices available to assist people who are recovering from or adapting to a physical condition.

_____

5. Its purpose is to help with balance. Residents using one of these should be able to bear weight on both legs.

_____

Down

2. Adaptive equipment is designed to assist the resident while doing these.

_____

3. These are used for residents who can bear no weight or limited weight on one leg.

_____

Unit 4: Describe positioning and how to assist with range of motion (ROM) exercises

Labeling.

Label each position below correctly.

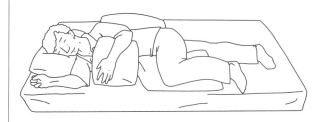

1. _____

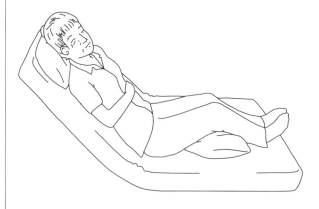

2. _____

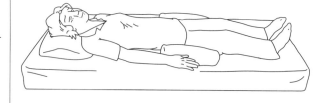

3. _____

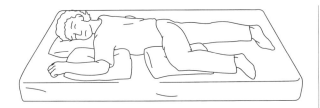

4. _____

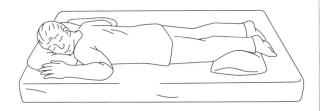

5. _____

Matching.

Write the letter of the correct definition beside each term listed below.

a. turning downward

b. moving a body part toward the body

c. turning upward

d. bending backward

e. moving a body part away from the body

f. straightening a body part

g. bending a body part

h. turning a joint

6. _____ abduction

7. _____ adduction

8. _____ dorsiflexion

9. _____ rotation

10. _____ extension

11. _____ flexion

12. _____ pronation

13. _____ supination

Labeling.

Correctly label each of the following movements used in range of motion exercises.

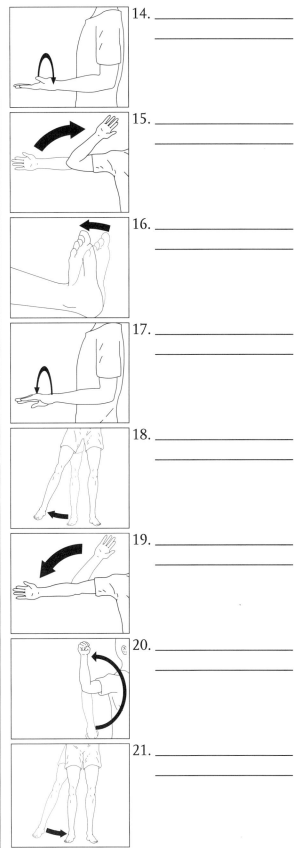

14. _____
_____

15. _____
_____

16. _____
_____

17. _____
_____

18. _____
_____

19. _____
_____

20. _____
_____

21. _____
_____

Name: _____

Unit 5: List guidelines for assisting with bowel and bladder retraining

Scenarios.

Read the following paragraphs and answer the questions.

Patty, a nursing assistant, sees that a resident has been incontinent. She says, "Oh no! You were doing so well until now."

1. What is wrong with Patty's reaction?

_____

_____

_____

_____

_____

Tom, a nursing assistant, knows that a resident was incontinent last night. The resident asks Tom for a drink. Tom tells him, "You can't have any water now or you might have another accident."

2. What is wrong with Tom's reaction?

_____

_____

_____

_____

_____

Jesse, a nursing assistant, enters a resident's room and begins giving her a long massage before bed. At the end of the massage, Jesse notices urine on the sheets.

3. What could Jesse have done that might have prevented this?

_____

_____

_____

_____

_____

_____

Celia enters a resident's room and asks, "Is it time to change your diaper now?"

4. What is wrong with what Celia said?

_____

_____

_____

_____

_____

Unit 6: Describe care and use of prosthetic devices

True or False.

Mark each statement with either a "T" for true or "F" for false.

1. _____ A prosthesis may replace an eye, arm, hand, foot, or leg.

2. _____ If you see that a prosthesis is cracked, try to repair it yourself.

3. _____ Prostheses are very expensive.

4. _____ A resident with a prosthesis will need special attention to help him adjust to changes.

5. _____ You will be responsible for assisting a resident with a prosthesis with ADLs and ambulation.

6. _____ You should report any redness or open areas that a resident with a prosthesis has.

7. _____ It is not important to keep a prosthesis clean and dry.

8. _____ If the way a stump looks bothers you, you should tell the resident this.

TEN

Caring for Yourself

Unit 1: Describe how to find a great job

Word Search.

Complete each of the following sentences and find your answers in the word search.

i	e	s	u	p	e	r	v	i	s	o	r	d	d
e	d	y	n	e	a	t	l	y	g	u	f	y	y
u	p	e	e	j	p	h	l	i	n	c	a	c	h
r	o	c	n	s	u	a	l	c	y	o	i	r	h
s	s	x	j	t	r	i	h	u	j	v	e	a	d
e	i	u	z	h	i	u	z	a	x	i	p	n	r
c	t	p	a	n	i	f	o	a	l	p	u	g	f
n	i	f	v	h	g	j	i	h	y	o	o	y	y
e	v	j	a	i	l	s	e	c	r	l	b	c	a
r	e	g	j	w	d	h	e	g	a	d	a	y	k
e	u	c	t	z	z	l	k	q	g	t	c	p	d
f	v	y	y	o	I	c	c	s	s	c	i	c	k
e	s	d	t	m	a	t	u	p	b	w	q	o	z
r	w	c	s	b	n	u	t	c	d	n	l	h	n

1. You should bring _____ *identification* with you to a job interview, such as a driver's license, social security card, passport, or birth certificate.

2. When arriving at a job interview, introduce yourself, _____, and shake hands.

3. _____ are people who can be called to recommend you as an employee.

4. Never _____ *lie* on a job application.

5. Be _____ *positive* when answering any questions during a job interview.

6. By law, your employer must perform a criminal _____ check. It is a law intended to protect residents.

7. Make sure you are dressed _____ and appropriately for a job interview.

8. During a job interview make _____ contact to show you are sincere.

9. Sit up or stand up straight, and look _____ to be at a job interview.

10. Questions you may want to ask during an interview include: How much contact would I have with my _____ and what _____ would I work?

Short Answer.

11. Look at the illustration on the next page. This person is going to a job interview. What are some examples of how she appears unprofessional?

_____

_____

Name: _____

_____
_____
_____
_____

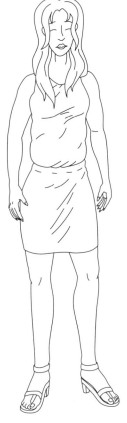

Unit 2: Describe ways to be a great employee

Samantha is a nursing assistant at Rolling Meadows Nursing Home. During one of her shifts, Samantha is called into her supervisor's office. Her supervisor says, "I've noticed that you've been late to work three times in a row. It's not fair to the other nursing assistants. And yesterday, you were unable to finish your assigned care tasks before your shift ended."

Samantha says, "I'm sorry I've been late. I've had a difficult time getting my son ready for school in the mornings. I'll make more of an effort to be on time. I know it's not fair to the others."

1. In this situation, what did Samantha do correctly?

_____
_____
_____
_____
_____
_____
_____
_____

Jamie, a nursing assistant, walks into Mrs. Sandoval's room. Mrs. Sandoval's son and daughter are visiting her. When Jamie enters, Mrs. Sandoval's son walks over to her and yells, "It took you long enough to get here! My mother rang her call light ten minutes ago. Are you too busy taking a break to get in here?"

Jamie says, "I got here as fast as I could. Why don't you just help her yourself if I'm so slow?"

2. In this situation, what did Jamie do incorrectly?

_____
_____
_____
_____
_____
_____
_____
_____

Unit 3: Review guidelines for behaving professionally on the job

Mark a "P" next to all the examples of professional behavior.

1. _____ Showing up for your shift 15 minutes late

2. _____ Wearing a uniform that has a stain on it

3. _____ Keeping your nails clean and trimmed

4. _____ Washing your hair and tying it back neatly

5. _____ Telling a resident that you enjoy spending time with him

6. _____ Not calling into work when you're sick

7. _____ Reporting a resident's new rash to the nurse

8. _____ Telling your supervisor, "I don't understand what that means. Can you please explain it?"

9. _____ Explaining a procedure to a resident before performing it

10. _____ Not telling another nursing assistant that a resident was in pain this morning

11. _____ Suggesting to your supervisor that you could take an agitated resident for a walk

Unit 4: Describe continuing education for nursing assistants

True or False.

Mark each statement with either a "T" for true or "F" for false.

1. _____ The federal government requires 20 hours of continuing education each year.

2. _____ Each state maintains a registry for certified nursing assistants (CNAs).

3. _____ Your responsibility for in-service education is to successfully attend and complete classes.

4. _____ Some states require more continuing education than the federal government.

5 _____ In-service continuing education courses help you keep your knowledge fresh.

Short Answer.

6. List four of the responsibilities nursing assistants have for receiving continuing education.

_____

_____

_____

_____

_____

_____

_____

_____

_____

_____

_____

_____

_____

_____

Unit 5: Define stress and discuss ways to manage it

Multiple Choice.

Circle the letter of the answer that best completes the statement.

1. Stress is a _____ response.

   a. relaxation

   b. emotional

   c. physical

   d. both b and c

Name: _____

2. When your heart beats fast in stressful situations, it can be a result of an increase of the hormone:

    a. testosterone

    b. estrogen

    c. adrenaline

    d. progesterone

3. Not managing your stress can cause:

    a. arguments

    b. fatigue

    c. abusive behavior

    d. all of the above

4. A healthy body is the result of:

    a. eating when you're not hungry

    b. exercising regularly

    c. drinking moderately

    d. none of the above

5. When you're stressed, you can turn to the following for help:

    a. your residents

    b. your supervisor

    c. your residents' family members

    d. all of the above

Short Answer.

1. What are some of the things that make you experience stress? How do you react when you're stressed?

    _____

    _____

    _____

    _____

    _____

    _____

    _____

    _____

2. Write out your own personal stress management plan. Be sure to include things like diet, exercise, relaxation, exercise, entertainment, etc.

    _____

    _____

    _____

    _____

    _____

    _____

    _____

    _____

    _____

    _____

    _____

PROCEDURE CHECKLISTS

Many skills evaluations during certification exams list washing your hands as the final step to perform. Although you will not necessarily be tested on documenting a procedure or reporting changes to the nurse during a certification exam, those final steps are included in these procedure checklists. These steps are important. In a facility, you will need to document every procedure you perform. You will also need to report any changes you notice while providing care.

TWO

Foundations of Resident Care

Heimlich Maneuver for the Conscious Person

✓ **Procedure Steps**

☐ 1. Stands behind person and brings arms under person's arms. Wraps arms around person's waist.

☐ 2. Makes a fist with one hand. Places flat, thumb side of the fist against person's abdomen, above the navel but below the breastbone.

☐ 3. Grasps the fist with other hand. Pulls both hands toward self and up, quickly and forcefully.

☐ 4. Repeats until object is pushed out or person loses consciousness.

Comments:

Heimlich Maneuver for the Unconscious Person

✓ **Procedure Steps**

☐ 1. Makes sure person is on his back.

☐ 2. Opens the airway by tilting head back and lifting the chin.

☐ 3. Checks for breath.

☐ 4. If there is no breathing, opens the mouth and sweeps mouth with finger to remove blockage. Sweeps along the inside of the mouth toward the base of the tongue.

☐ 5. Pinches the nose closed and gives two full breaths.

☐ 6. If air still does not enter the airway, kneels and straddles person's thighs, facing his face.

☐ 7. Places the heel of one hand on person's abdomen, slightly above the navel, with fingers pointing toward person's chest. Places other hand over the first hand.

☐ 8. Gives five abdominal thrusts by pushing hands inward and upward.

☐ 9. Checks to see if blockage is removed.

☐ 10. Tries to sweep the object out with fingers.

☐ 11. Repeat steps if necessary.

Comments:

Shock

✓ **Procedure Steps**

- ❏ 1. Has the person lie down on her back unless bleeding from the mouth or vomiting.
- ❏ 2. Controls bleeding if bleeding occurs.
- ❏ 3. Checks pulse and respirations if possible.
- ❏ 4. Keeps person as calm and comfortable as possible.
- ❏ 5. Maintains normal body temperature.
- ❏ 6. Elevates the feet unless person has a head or abdominal injury, breathing difficulties, or a fractured bone or back.
- ❏ 7. Does not give person anything to eat or drink.
- ❏ 8. Calls for help immediately.

Comments:

Heart Attack

✓ **Procedure Steps**

- ❏ 1. Calls or has someone call the nurse.
- ❏ 2. Places person in a comfortable position. Encourages him to rest, and reassures him that he will not be left alone.
- ❏ 3. Loosens clothing around the neck.
- ❏ 4. Does not give person liquids.
- ❏ 5. If person takes heart medication, such as nitroglycerin, finds medication and offers it to him. Does not place medication in person's mouth.
- ❏ 6. Monitors person's breathing and pulse. If breathing stops or person

has no pulse, performs rescue breathing or CPR if trained to do so.

- ❏ 7. Stays with person until help arrives.

Comments:

Fainting

✓ **Procedure Steps**

- ❏ 1. Has person lie down or sit down before fainting occurs.
- ❏ 2. If person is in sitting position, has him bend forward and place his head between his knees. If person is lying flat on his back, elevates the legs.
- ❏ 3. Reports the incident to the nurse.
- ❏ 4. Loosens any tight clothing.
- ❏ 5. Has person stay in position for at least five minutes after symptoms disappear.
- ❏ 6. Helps person get up slowly. Continues to observe him for symptoms of fainting.

Comments:

Seizures

✓ **Procedure Steps**

- ❏ 1. Lowers person to the floor.
- ❏ 2. Has someone call the nurse immediately. Does not leave person unless has to get medical help.
- ❏ 3. Moves furniture away to prevent injury. If a pillow is nearby, places it under his head.
- ❏ 4. Does not try to restrain the person.

❏ 5. Does not force anything between the person's teeth. Does not place hands in person's mouth.

❏ 6. Does not give liquids.

❏ 7. When the seizure is over, checks breathing.

❏ 8. Reports the length of the seizure and observations to the nurse.

Comments:

Bleeding

✓ **Procedure Steps**

❏ 1. Puts on gloves.

❏ 2. Holds thick sterile pad or a clean cloth against the wound.

❏ 3. Presses down hard directly on the bleeding wound until help arrives. Does not decrease pressure. Puts additional pads over the first pad if blood seeps through. Does not remove the first pad.

❏ 4. Raises the wound above the heart to slow down the bleeding.

❏ 5. When bleeding is under control, secures the dressing to keep it in place. Checks person for symptoms of shock. Stays with person until help arrives.

❏ 6. Washes hands.

Comments:

Washing hands

✓ **Procedure Steps**

❏ 1. Turns on water at sink.

❏ 2. Angles arms down holding hands lower than elbows. Wets hands and wrists thoroughly.

❏ 3. Applies skin cleanser or soap to hands.

❏ 4. Lathers all surfaces of fingers and hands, including above the wrists, producing friction, for at least 10 seconds.

❏ 5. Cleans nails by rubbing them in palm of other hand.

❏ 6. Rinses all surfaces of hands and wrists, running water down from wrists to fingertips.

❏ 7. Uses clean, dry paper towel to dry all surfaces of hands, wrists, and fingers.

❏ 8. Uses clean, dry paper towel or clean, dry area of paper towel to turn off faucet, without contaminating hands.

❏ 9. Disposes of used paper towel(s) in wastebasket immediately after shutting off faucet.

Comments:

Putting on gloves

✓ **Procedure Steps**

❏ 1. Washes hands.

❏ 2. If right-handed, slides one glove on left hand (reverse, if left-handed).

❏ 3. With gloved hand takes second glove and slides other hand into the glove.

❏ 4. Interlaces fingers to smooth out folds and create a comfortable fit.

☐ 5. Carefully looks for tears, holes, or spots. Replaces the glove if necessary.

☐ 6. If wearing a gown, pulls the cuff of the gloves over the sleeve of gown.

Comments:

Taking off gloves

✓ **Procedure Steps**

☐ 1. Touches only the outside of one glove and pulls the first glove off, turning it inside out.

☐ 2. With ungloved hand, reaches two fingers inside the remaining glove. Does not touch any part of the outside.

☐ 3. Pulls down, turning this glove inside out and over the first glove.

☐ 4. Disposes of gloves properly.

☐ 5. Washes hands.

Comments:

Putting on a gown

✓ **Procedure Steps**

☐ 1. Washes hands.

☐ 2. Opens gown without shaking it. Slips arms into the sleeves and pulls gown on.

☐ 3. Ties neck ties.

☐ 4. Pulls gown until it completely covers clothing. Ties the back ties.

Comments:

Putting on a mask and eye shield

✓ **Procedure Steps**

☐ 1. Washes hands.

☐ 2. Picks up mask by top strings or elastic strap. Does not touch mask where it touches face.

☐ 3. Adjusts mask over nose and mouth. Ties top strings first, then bottom string.

☐ 4. Puts on eye shield.

Comments:

FIVE

Personal Care Skills

Giving a complete bed bath

✓ **Procedure Steps**

☐ 1. Washes hands.

☐ 2. Identifies self to resident by name. Addresses resident by name.

☐ 3. Explains procedure to resident, speaking clearly, slowly, and directly, maintaining face-to-face contact whenever possible.

☐ 4. Provides for resident's privacy during procedure with curtain, screen, or door.

☐ 5. Adjusts bed to a safe working level.

☐ 6. Adjusts position of side rails throughout procedure to ensure resident safety at all times.

☐ 7. Removes or folds back top bedding, keeping resident covered with bath blanket (or top sheet).

❑ 8. Tests water temperature with thermometer or wrist. Water temperature should be 110° to 115° F. Has resident check water temperature. Adjusts if necessary.

❑ 9. Puts on gloves if resident has open lesions or wounds.

❑ 10. Asks and assists resident to participate in washing.

❑ 11. Uncovers only one part of the body at a time. Places a towel under the body part being washed.

❑ 12. Washes, rinses, and dries one part of the body at a time. Starts at the head, working down, and completing front first.

Eyes and Face:

❑ Washes face with wet washcloth (no soap) beginning with the eyes, using a different area of the washcloth for each eye, washing inner aspect to outer aspect. Washes the face from the middle outward using firm but gentle strokes. Washes neck and ears and behind the ears. Rinses and pats dry.

Arms:

❑ Washes arm and underarm. Uses long strokes from the shoulder down to the elbow. Rinses and pats dry. Washes the elbow. Washes, rinses, and dries from the elbow down to the wrist. Washes hand in a basin. Provides nail care if it has been assigned.

Chest and Abdomen:

❑ Washes, rinses, and pats dry, only uncovering one part at a time. For a female resident: washes, rinses, and dries breasts and under breasts.

Legs:

❑ Washes the thigh. Uses long downward strokes. Rinses and pats dry. Does the same from the knee to the ankle.

❑ Washes the foot and between the toes in a basin. Rinses foot and pats dry. Provides nail care if it has been assigned.

Back:

❑ Helps resident move to the center of the bed, then turns onto his side so back is facing self. Washes back, neck, and buttocks with long, downward strokes. Rinses and pats dry.

❑ 13. Puts on gloves before washing perineal area.

❑ 14. Changes bath water. Washes, rinses, and dries perineal area, working from front to back.

For a female resident:

❑ Washes the perineum with soap and water from front to back, using single strokes. Uses a clean area of washcloth or clean washcloth for each stroke. Wipes the center of the perineum, then each side. Spreads the labia majora, the outside folds of perineal skin that protect the urinary meatus and the vaginal opening. Wipes from front to back on each side. Rinses the area in the same way. Dries entire perineal area moving from front to back, using a blotting motion with towel. Asks resident to turn on her side. Washes, rinses, and dries buttocks and anal area. Cleanses anal area without contaminating the perineal area.

For a male resident:

❑ If resident is uncircumcised, retracts the foreskin first. Gently pushes skin towards the base of penis.

❑ Holds the penis by the shaft and washes in a circular motion from the tip down to the base. Uses a clean area of washcloth or clean washcloth for each stroke. Rinses the penis. Then washes the scrotum and groin. Rinses and pats dry. If resident is uncircumcised, gently returns foreskin to normal position. Asks resident to turn on his side. Washes, rinses, and dries buttocks and anal area. Cleanses anal area without contaminating the perineal area.

❑ 15. Applies lotion and deodorant. Does not apply lotion between the toes.

❑ 16. Removes and disposes of gloves properly.

❑ 17. Puts clean gown on resident. Assists resident to a position of safety and comfort and replaces bedding.

❑ 18. Returns bed to appropriate level. Puts signaling device within resident's reach.

❑ 19. Places soiled clothing and linens in appropriate containers.

❑ 20. Empties, rinses, and wipes bath basin and returns to proper storage.

❑ 21. Washes hands.

❑ 22. Reports any changes in resident.

❑ 23. Documents procedure.

Comments:

Shampooing in bed

✓ Procedure Steps

❑ 1. Washes hands.

❑ 2. Identifies self to resident by name. Addresses resident by name.

❑ 3. Explains procedure to resident, speaking clearly, slowly, and directly, maintaining face-to-face contact whenever possible.

❑ 4. Provides for resident's privacy during procedure with curtain, screen, or door.

❑ 5. Adjusts bed to a safe working level. Removes pillow.

❑ 6. Tests water temperature with thermometer or wrist. Water temperature should be 110° to 115° F. Has resident check water temperature. Adjusts if necessary.

❑ 7. Raises the side rail farthest from self.

❑ 8. Places the waterproof pad underneath resident's head and shoulders.

❑ 9. Places collection container under resident's head (e.g., trough, basin). Places one towel across resident's shoulders.

❑ 10. Protects resident's eyes with dry washcloth.

❑ 11. Wets hair and applies shampoo.

❑ 12. Lathers and massages scalp with fingertips without scratching scalp.

❑ 13. Rinses hair until water runs clear. Applies conditioner and rinses as directed.

❑ 14. Covers resident's hair with clean towel. Dries face with washcloth.

❑ 15. Removes trough and waterproof covering.

❑ 16. Raises head of bed.

❑ 17. Gently rubs the scalp and hair with the towel.

❑ 18. Dries and combs resident's hair according to resident's preference.

❑ 19. Returns bed to appropriate level.

❑ 20. Puts signaling device within resident's reach.

❑ 21. Empties, rinses, and wipes bath basin/pitcher and returns to proper storage.

❑ 22. Cleans comb/brush and returns hairdryer and comb/brush to proper storage.

❑ 23. Places soiled linen in soiled linen container.

❑ 24. Washes hands.

❑ 25. Reports any changes in resident.

❑ 26. Documents procedure.

Comments:

Giving a shower

✓ Procedure Steps

❑ 1. Washes hands.

❑ 2. Identifies self to resident by name. Addresses resident by name.

❑ 3. Explains procedure to resident, speaking clearly, slowly, and directly, maintaining face-to-face contact whenever possible.

❑ 4. Provides for resident's privacy during procedure with curtain, screen, or door.

❑ 5. Cleans shower area and shower chair.

❑ 6. Places shower chair into position and locks wheels. Safely transfers resident into shower chair.

❑ 7. Turns on water. Tests water temperature with thermometer. Water temperature should be no more than 105° F. Has resident check water temperature.

❑ 8. Puts on gloves.

❑ 9. Helps resident remove clothing. Drapes resident with bath blanket.

❑ 10. Stays with resident during procedure.

❑ 11. Pushes shower chair into shower.

❑ 12. Lets resident wash as much as possible. Assists to wash the face.

❑ 13. Helps resident shampoo and rinse hair.

❑ 14. Assists to wash and rinse the entire body, moving from head to toe.

❑ 15. Turns off water. Rolls resident out of shower.

❑ 16. Gives resident towel(s) and assists to pat dry. Pats dry under the breasts, between skin folds, in the perineal area, and between toes.

❑ 17. Places soiled clothing and linens in appropriate containers.

❑ 18. Applies lotion and deodorant.

❑ 19. Removes gloves and washes hands.

❑ 20. Helps resident dress and comb hair and return to room.

❑ 21. Places signaling device within resident's reach.

❑ 22. Reports any changes in resident.

❑ 23. Documents procedure.

Comments:

Providing fingernail care

✓ Procedure Steps

❑ 1. Washes hands.

❑ 2. Identifies self to resident by name. Addresses resident by name.

❑ 3. Explains procedure to resident, speaking clearly, slowly, and directly, maintaining face-to-face contact whenever possible.

❑ 4. Provides for resident's privacy during procedure with curtain, screen, or door.

❑ 5. Adjusts bed to a safe working level.

❑ 6. Tests water temperature with thermometer or wrist. Water temperature should be 110° to 115° F. Has resident check water temperature. Adjusts if necessary.

❑ 7. Immerses resident's hands in basin of water. Soaks hands for two to four minutes.

❑ 8. Removes hands. Washes hands with soapy washcloth. Rinses. Pats hands dry with towel, including between fingers.

❑ 9. Cleans under nails with orangewood stick.

❑ 10. Wipes orangewood stick on towel after each nail.

❑ 11. Grooms nails with file or emery board. Files in a curve.

❑ 12. Finishes with nails smooth and free of rough edges.

❑ 13. Applies lotion from fingertips to wrist.

❑ 14. Returns bed to appropriate level.

❑ 15. Places signaling device within resident's reach.

❑ 16. Empties, rinses, and wipes basin, and returns to proper storage.

❑ 17. Disposes of soiled linen in the soiled linen container.

❑ 18. Washes hands.

❑ 19. Reports any changes in resident.

❑ 20. Documents procedure.

Comments:

Providing foot care

✓ **Procedure Steps**

❑ 1. Washes hands.

❑ 2. Identifies self to resident by name. Addresses resident by name.

❑ 3. Explains procedure to resident, speaking clearly, slowly, and directly, maintaining face-to-face contact whenever possible.

❑ 4. Provides for resident's privacy during procedure with curtain, screen, or door.

❑ 5. Adjusts bed to a safe working level.

❑ 6. Tests water temperature with thermometer or wrist. Water temperature should be 105° F. Has resident check water temperature. Adjusts if necessary.

❑ 7. Places basin on the bath mat.

❑ 8. Removes socks. Completely submerges feet in water. Soaks feet for five to ten minutes.

❑ 9. Removes one foot from water. Washes entire foot, including between the toes and around nail beds, with soapy washcloth.

❑ 10. Rinses entire foot, including between the toes.

❑ 11. Dries entire foot, including between the toes.

❑ 12. Repeats steps for the other foot.

❑ 13. Puts lotion in hand and warms it by rubbing hands together.

❑ 14. Massages lotion into entire foot, removing any excess with a towel.

❑ 15. Assists resident to replace socks.

❑ 16. Returns bed to appropriate level.

❑ 17. Places signaling device within resident's reach.

❑ 18. Empties, rinses, and wipes basin, and returns to proper storage.

❑ 19. Disposes of soiled linen in the soiled linen container.

❑ 20. Washes hands.

❑ 21. Reports any changes in resident.

❑ 22. Documents procedure.

Comments:

Combing or brushing hair

✓ Procedure Steps

❑ 1. Washes hands.

❑ 2. Identifies self to resident by name. Addresses resident by name.

❑ 3. Explains procedure to resident, speaking clearly, slowly, and directly, maintaining face-to-face contact whenever possible.

❑ 4. Provides for resident's privacy during procedure with curtain, screen, or door.

❑ 5. Raises head of bed so resident is sitting up. Places a towel under head or around shoulders.

❑ 6. Removes any hair pins, hair ties, and clips.

❑ 7. Removes tangles. Gently combs out from ends of hair to scalp.

❑ 8. Brushes two-inch sections of hair at a time. Brushes from roots to ends.

❑ 9. Styles hair in the way resident prefers.

Avoids childish hairstyles. Offers mirror to resident.

❑ 10. Returns bed to appropriate level.

❑ 11. Places signaling device within resident's reach.

❑ 12. Returns supplies to proper storage. Cleans hair from brush/comb.

❑ 13. Disposes of soiled linen in the soiled linen container.

❑ 14. Washes hands.

❑ 15. Reports any changes in resident.

❑ 16. Documents procedure.

Comments:

Shaving a resident

✓ Procedure Steps

❑ 1. Washes hands.

❑ 2. Identifies self to resident by name. Addresses resident by name.

❑ 3. Explains procedure to resident, speaking clearly, slowly, and directly, maintaining face-to-face contact whenever possible.

❑ 4. Provides for resident's privacy during procedure with curtain, screen, or door.

❑ 5. Raises head of bed so resident is sitting up.

Shaving using a safety razor:

❑ 6. Fills basin halfway with warm water and drapes towel under resident's chin.

❑ 7. Applies gloves.

❑ 8. Moistens beard with warm washcloth. Puts shaving cream or soap over area.

❑ 9. Holds skin taut and shaves beard in downward strokes on face and upward strokes on neck. Rinses razor often in warm water.

❑ 10. Offers mirror to resident.

❑ 11. Washes, rinses, and dries face after the shave. Applies after-shave lotion as requested.

❑ 12. Removes towel.

❑ 13. Removes gloves.

Shaving using an electric razor:

❑ 6. Drapes towel under resident's chin.

❑ 7. Applies gloves.

❑ 8. Applies pre-shave lotion as resident wishes.

❑ 9. Holds skin taut. Shaves with smooth, even movements.

❑ 10. Offers mirror to resident.

❑ 11. Applies after-shave lotion as requested.

❑ 12. Removes towel.

❑ 13. Removes gloves.

Final steps:

❑ 14. Makes sure that resident and environment are free of loose hairs.

❑ 15. Returns bed to appropriate level.

❑ 16. Places signaling device within resident's reach.

❑ 17. For safety razor: Rinses safety razor. For disposable razor: Disposes of a disposable razor in appropriate biohazard container. For electric razor: Cleans head of electric razor. Removes whiskers from razor. Recaps shaving head. Returns razor to case.

❑ 18. Returns supplies and equipment to proper storage.

❑ 19. Washes hands.

❑ 20. Reports any changes in resident.

❑ 21. Documents procedure.

Comments:

Providing mouth care

✓ **Procedure Steps**

❑ 1. Washes hands.

❑ 2. Identifies self to resident by name. Addresses resident by name.

❑ 3. Explains procedure to resident, speaking clearly, slowly, and directly, maintaining face-to-face contact whenever possible.

❑ 4. Provides for resident's privacy during procedure with curtain, screen, or door.

❑ 5. Adjusts bed to a safe working level. Makes sure resident is in an upright sitting position.

❑ 6. Puts on gloves.

❑ 7. Places towel across resident's chest.

❑ 8. Wets brush and puts on small amount of toothpaste.

❑ 9. Cleans entire mouth (including tongue and all surfaces of teeth), using gentle motions. First brushes upper teeth, then lower teeth.

❑ 10. Holds emesis basin to resident's chin.

❑ 11. Has resident rinse mouth with water and spit into emesis basin.

❑ 12. Wipes resident's mouth and removes towel.

❑ 13. Disposes of soiled linen in the soiled linen container.

❑ 14. Cleans and returns supplies to proper storage.

❑ 15. Removes gloves. Disposes of gloves properly.

❑ 16. Returns bed to appropriate level.

❑ 17. Places signaling device within resident's reach.

❑ 18. Washes hands.

❑ 19. Reports any problems with teeth, mouth, tongue, and lips.

❑ 20. Documents procedure.

Comments:

Flossing teeth

✓ **Procedure Steps**

❑ 1. Washes hands.

❑ 2. Identifies self to resident by name. Addresses resident by name.

❑ 3. Explains procedure to resident, speaking clearly, slowly, and directly, maintaining face-to-face contact whenever possible.

❑ 4. Provides for resident's privacy during procedure with curtain, screen, or door.

❑ 5. Adjusts the bed to a safe working level. Makes sure resident is in an upright sitting position.

❑ 6. Puts on gloves.

❑ 7. Wraps the ends of floss securely around each index finger.

❑ 8. Starting with the back teeth, places floss between teeth and moves it down the surface of the tooth using a gentle sawing motion. Continues to the gum line. At the gum line, curves the floss into a letter C, slips it gently into the space between the gum and tooth, then goes back up, scraping that side of the tooth.

❑ 9. Repeats this on the side of the other tooth.

❑ 10. After every two or three teeth, unwinds floss from fingers and moves it so clean area is used. Flosses all teeth.

❑ 11. Offers water to rinse debris from the mouth into the basin.

❑ 12. Offers resident a face towel when done flossing all teeth.

❑ 13. Disposes of soiled linen in the soiled linen container.

❑ 14. Cleans and returns supplies to proper storage.

❑ 15. Removes and disposes of gloves properly.

❑ 16. Returns bed to appropriate level.

❑ 17. Places signaling device within resident's reach.

❑ 18. Washes hands.

❑ 19. Reports any problems with teeth, mouth, tongue, and lips.

❑ 20. Documents procedure.

Comments:

Cleaning and storing dentures

✓ **Procedure Steps**

❑ 1. Washes hands.

❑ 2. Puts on gloves.

❑ 3. Lines sink/basin with a towel(s).

❑ 4. Rinses dentures in cool running water before brushing them.

❏ 5. Applies toothpaste or cleanser to toothbrush.

❏ 6. Brushes dentures on all surfaces.

❏ 7. Rinses all surfaces of dentures under cool running water.

❏ 8. Rinses denture cup before placing clean dentures in it.

❏ 9. Places dentures in clean denture cup with solution or cool water. Makes sure cup is labeled with resident's name.

❏ 10. Cleans and returns the equipment to proper storage.

❏ 11. Disposes of towels in appropriate container.

❏ 12. Removes gloves. Disposes of gloves properly.

❏ 13. Washes hands.

❏ 14. Reports any changes in appearance of dentures.

❏ 15. Documents procedure.

Comments:

Providing mouth care for the unconscious resident

✓ **Procedure Steps**

❏ 1. Washes hands.

❏ 2. Identifies self to resident by name. Addresses resident by name.

❏ 3. Explains procedure to resident, speaking clearly, slowly, and directly, maintaining face-to-face contact whenever possible.

❏ 4. Provides for resident's privacy during procedure with curtain, screen, or door.

❏ 5. Adjusts bed to a safe working level.

❏ 6. Puts on gloves.

❏ 7. Turns resident's head to the side and places a towel under his cheek and chin. Places an emesis basin next to the cheek and chin.

❏ 8. Holds mouth open with padded tongue blade.

❏ 9. Dips swab in cleaning solution. Wipes teeth, gums, tongue, and inside surfaces of mouth, changing swab frequently. Repeats until the mouth is clean.

❏ 10. Rinses with clean swab dipped in water.

❏ 11. Removes the towel and basin. Pats lips or face dry if needed. Applies lip moisturizer.

❏ 12. Disposes of soiled linen in the soiled linen container.

❏ 13. Cleans and returns supplies to proper storage.

❏ 14. Removes gloves. Disposes of gloves properly.

❏ 15. Returns bed to appropriate level.

❏ 16. Places signaling device within resident's reach.

❏ 17. Washes hands.

❏ 18. Reports any changes in resident.

❏ 19. Documents procedure.

Comments:

Dressing a resident with an affected right arm

✓ **Procedure Steps**

❏ 1. Washes hands.

2. Identifies self to resident by name. Addresses resident by name.

3. Explains procedure to resident, speaking clearly, slowly, and directly, maintaining face-to-face contact whenever possible.

4. Provides for resident's privacy during procedure with curtain, screen, or door.

5. Asks resident which outfit she would like to wear. Dresses her in outfit of choice.

6. Removes resident's gown without completely exposing resident. Takes off stronger side first when undressing.

7. Assists resident to put the right (affected) arm through the right sleeve of the shirt, sweater, or slip before placing garment on left (unaffected) arm.

8. Assists resident to put on skirt, pants, or dress.

9. Places bed at a safe and appropriate level for resident, usually the lowest position.

10. Applies non-skid footwear.

11. Puts on all items, moving resident's body gently and naturally, avoiding force and over-extension of limbs and joints.

12. Finishes with resident dressed appropriately. Makes sure clothing is right-side-out and zippers/buttons are fastened.

13. Places gown in soiled linen container.

14. Places signaling device within resident's reach.

15. Washes hands.

16. Reports any changes in resident.

17. Documents procedure.

Comments:

Assisting resident with use of bedpan

✓ **Procedure Steps**

1. Washes hands.

2. Identifies self to resident by name. Addresses resident by name.

3. Explains procedure to resident, speaking clearly, slowly, and directly, maintaining face-to-face contact whenever possible.

4. Provides for resident's privacy during procedure with curtain, screen, or door.

5. Applies gloves.

6. Before placing bedpan, lowers head of bed.

7. Places a protective pad under resident's buttocks and hips.

8. Asks resident to remove undergarments or help him do so.

9. Places bedpan correctly under resident's buttocks (Standard bedpan: Positions bedpan so wider end of pan is aligned with resident's buttocks; Fracture pan: Positions bedpan with handle toward foot of bed).

10. Raises head of bed after placing bedpan under resident.

11. Puts toilet tissue within resident's reach.

12. Leaves signaling device within resident's reach while resident is using bedpan. Asks resident to signal when finished.

❏ 13. Returns and lowers head of bed.

❏ 14. Removes bedpan carefully. Covers bedpan.

❏ 15. Provides perineal care if assistance is needed.

❏ 16. Empties contents of bedpan into toilet. Notes color, odor, and consistency of contents.

❏ 17. Rinses bedpan, pouring rinse water into toilet, and returns to proper storage.

❏ 18. Removes and disposes of gloves properly.

❏ 19. Assists resident to wash hands. Disposes of soiled washcloth or wipes in proper container. Helps resident put on undergarment.

❏ 20. Returns bed to appropriate level.

❏ 21. Places signaling device within resident's reach.

❏ 22. Washes hands.

❏ 23. Reports any changes in resident.

❏ 24. Documents procedure.

Comments:

Assisting a male resident with a urinal

✓ Procedure Steps

❏ 1. Washes hands.

❏ 2. Identifies self to resident by name. Addresses resident by name.

❏ 3. Explains procedure to resident, speaking clearly, slowly, and directly, maintaining face-to-face contact whenever possible.

❏ 4. Provides for resident's privacy during procedure with curtain, screen, or door.

❏ 5. Applies gloves.

❏ 6. Places a protective pad under resident's buttocks and hips.

❏ 7. Hands the urinal to resident. If resident is not able to help himself, places urinal between his legs and positions penis inside the urinal. Replaces bed covers.

❏ 8. Leaves signaling device within resident's reach. Asks resident to signal when finished.

❏ 9. Removes urinal; empties contents into toilet. Notes color, odor, and qualities of contents.

❏ 10. Rinses urinal, pouring rinse water into toilet, and returns to proper storage.

❏ 11. Removes and disposes of gloves.

❏ 12. Assists resident to wash hands. Disposes of soiled washcloth or wipes in proper container.

❏ 13. Places signaling device within resident's reach.

❏ 14. Washes hands.

❏ 15. Reports any changes in resident.

❏ 16. Documents procedure.

Comments:

Helping a resident use a portable commode

✓ Procedure Steps

❏ 1. Washes hands.

❏ 2. Identifies self to resident by name. Addresses resident by name.

❏ 3. Explains procedure to resident, speaking clearly, slowly, and directly, maintaining face-to-face contact whenever possible.

4. Provides for resident's privacy during procedure with curtain, screen, or door.

5. Helps to portable commode. Makes sure resident is wearing non-skid shoes.

6. If needed, helps resident remove clothing and sit comfortably on toilet seat. Puts toilet tissue within resident's reach.

7. Leaves signaling device within resident's reach. Asks resident to signal when finished.

8. Returns and applies gloves.

9. Provides perineal care if assistance is needed.

10. Assists resident to wash hands. Disposes of soiled washcloth or wipes in proper container.

11. Assists back to bed.

12. Removes waste container and empties contents into toilet. Notes color, odor, and consistency of contents.

13. Rinses container, pouring rinse water into toilet, and returns to proper storage.

14. After storing container, removes and disposes of gloves properly.

15. Places signaling device within resident's reach.

16. Washes hands.

17. Reports any changes in resident.

18. Documents procedure.

Comments:

Providing perineal care for incontinent resident

✓ Procedure Steps

1. Washes hands.

2. Identifies self to resident by name. Addresses resident by name.

3. Explains procedure to resident, speaking clearly, slowly, and directly, maintaining face-to-face contact whenever possible.

4. Provides for resident's privacy during procedure with curtain, screen, or door.

5. Adjusts bed to a safe working level.

6. Lowers head of bed. Positions resident lying flat on his or her back. Raises the side rail farthest from you.

7. Tests water temperature with thermometer or wrist. Water temperature should be 105° to 109° F. Has resident check water temperature. Adjusts if necessary.

8. Puts on gloves.

9. Removes soiled protective pad from underneath resident by turning resident on his side, away from self. Rolls soiled pad into itself with wet side in/dry side out.

10. Places clean protective pad under buttocks.

11. Returns resident to lying on his back.

12. Covers resident with bath blanket.

13. Exposes perineal area only. Cleans perineal area.

14. Turns resident on his side away from self. Removes the wet protective pad after drying buttocks.

15. Places a dry protective pad underneath resident.

❏ 16. Repositions resident.

❏ 17. Empties, rinses, and wipes basin and returns to proper storage.

❏ 18. Places soiled clothing and linens in appropriate containers.

❏ 19. Disposes of soiled protective pads in proper containers.

❏ 20. Removes and disposes of gloves properly.

❏ 21. Returns bed to appropriate level. Puts signaling device within resident's reach.

❏ 22. Washes hands.

❏ 23. Reports any changes in resident.

❏ 24. Documents procedure.

Comments:

Giving a back rub

✓ Procedure Steps

❏ 1. Washes hands.

❏ 2. Identifies self to resident by name. Addresses resident by name.

❏ 3. Explains procedure to resident, speaking clearly, slowly, and directly, maintaining face-to-face contact whenever possible.

❏ 4. Provides for resident's privacy during procedure with curtain, screen, or door.

❏ 5. Adjusts bed to a safe working level.

❏ 6. Positions resident lying on his stomach or on his side. Covers with a cotton blanket. Exposes back to the top of the buttocks.

❏ 7. Warms lotion.

❏ 8. Places hands on each side of upper part of the buttocks. Makes long, smooth upward strokes with both hands along each side of the spine, up to the shoulders Circles hands outward. Moves back along outer edges of the back. At buttocks, makes another circle and moves hands back up to the shoulders. Repeats this for three to five minutes without taking hands from resident's skin.

❏ 9. Makes kneading motions with the first two fingers and thumb of each hand. Places them at base of the spine. Moves upward together along each side of the spine, applying gentle downward pressure with fingers and thumbs. Follows same direction as with the long smooth strokes, circling at shoulders and buttocks.

❏ 10. Gently massages bony areas (spine, shoulder blades, hip bones) with circular motions of fingertips.

❏ 11. Finishes with some long, smooth strokes.

❏ 12. Dries the back if extra lotion remains on it.

❏ 13. Removes blanket and towel.

❏ 14. Assists resident with getting dressed.

❏ 15. Stores supplies. Places soiled clothing and linens in appropriate containers.

❏ 16. Returns bed to appropriate level.

❏ 17. Places signaling device within resident's reach.

❏ 18. Washes hands.

❏ 19. Reports any changes in resident.

❏ 20. Documents procedure.

Comments:

Name: _____

Assisting resident to move up in bed

✓ **Procedure Steps**

- ☐ 1. Washes hands.
- ☐ 2. Identifies self to resident by name. Addresses resident by name.
- ☐ 3. Explains procedure to resident, speaking clearly, slowly, and directly, maintaining face-to-face contact whenever possible.
- ☐ 4. Provides for resident's privacy during procedure with curtain, screen, or door.
- ☐ 5. Adjusts bed to a safe working level.
- ☐ 6. Lowers head of bed. Moves pillow to head of the bed. Locks bed wheels.
- ☐ 7. Lowers the side rail (if not already lowered) on side nearest self.
- ☐ 8. Stands alongside bed with feet apart, facing resident.
- ☐ 9. Places one arm under resident's shoulder blades and the other arm under resident's thighs.
- ☐ 10. Instructs resident to bend knees, brace feet on mattress, and push feet on the count of three.
- ☐ 11. On signal, shifts body weight to move resident, while resident pushes with her feet
- ☐ 12. Places pillow under resident's head.
- ☐ 13. Returns bed to appropriate level.
- ☐ 14. Places signaling device within resident's reach.
- ☐ 15. Washes hands.
- ☐ 16. Reports any changes in resident.
- ☐ 17. Documents procedure.

Comments:

Moving a resident to the side of the bed

✓ **Procedure Steps**

- ☐ 1. Washes hands.
- ☐ 2. Identifies self to resident by name. Addresses resident by name.
- ☐ 3. Explains procedure to resident, speaking clearly, slowly, and directly, maintaining face-to-face contact whenever possible.
- ☐ 4. Provides for resident's privacy during procedure with curtain, screen, or door.
- ☐ 5. Adjusts bed to a safe working level.
- ☐ 6. Lowers head of bed. Locks bed wheels.
- ☐ 7. Gently slides hands under the head and shoulders and moves toward self. Gently slides hands under midsection and moves toward self. Gently slides hands under hips and legs and moves toward self.
- ☐ 8. Returns bed to appropriate level.
- ☐ 9. Places signaling device within resident's reach.
- ☐ 10. Washes hands.
- ☐ 11. Reports any changes in resident.
- ☐ 12. Documents procedure.

Comments:

Turning a resident

✓ **Procedure Steps**

- ☐ 1. Washes hands.
- ☐ 2. Identifies self to resident by name. Addresses resident by name.

☐ 3. Explains procedure to resident, speaking clearly, slowly, and directly, maintaining face-to-face contact whenever possible.

☐ 4. Provides for resident's privacy during procedure with curtain, screen, or door.

☐ 5. Adjusts bed to a safe working level.

☐ 6. Lowers head of bed. Locks bed wheels.

☐ 7. Stands on side of bed opposite to where person will be turned. The far side rail should be raised.

☐ 8. Lowers side rail nearest self if it is up.

☐ 9. Moves resident to side of bed nearest self.

☐ 10. Crosses resident's arm over his or her chest. Crosses the leg nearest self over the far leg.

☐ 11. *Moving resident away from self:*

    a. Stands with feet approximately 12 inches apart. Bends knees.

    b. Places one hand on resident's shoulder and the other on resident's hip nearest self.

    c. Gently pushes resident toward the other side of the bed. Shifts weight from back leg to front leg.

☐   *Moving resident toward self:*

    a. Raises the side rail nearest self. Goes to the other side and lowers side rail.

    b. Stands with feet approximately 12 inches apart. Bends knees.

    c. Places one hand on resident's far shoulder and the other on resident's far hip.

    d. Gently rolls resident toward self.

☐ 12. Positions resident properly. Proper body alignment requires:

☐   head supported by pillow

☐   shoulder adjusted so resident is not lying on arm

☐   top arm supported by pillow

☐   back supported by supportive device

☐   top knee flexed

☐   top leg supported by supportive device with hip in proper alignment

☐ 13. Returns bed to appropriate level.

☐ 14. Places signaling device within resident's reach.

☐ 15. Washes hands.

☐ 16. Reports any changes in resident.

☐ 17. Documents procedure.

Comments:

Logrolling a resident with one assistant

✓ Procedure Steps

☐ 1. Washes hands.

☐ 2. Identifies self to resident by name. Addresses resident by name.

☐ 3. Explains procedure to resident, speaking clearly, slowly, and directly, maintaining face-to-face contact whenever possible.

☐ 4. Provides for resident's privacy during procedure with curtain, screen, or door.

☐ 5. Adjusts bed to a safe working level.

☐ 6. Lowers the head of bed. Locks bed wheels.

☐ 7. Lowers the side rail closest to self.

❑ 8. One person stands at resident's head and shoulders. The other stands near resident's midsection.

❑ 9. Places resident's arms across his or her chest. Places a pillow between the knees.

❑ 10. Stands with feet approximately 12 inches apart. Bends knees.

❑ 11. Grasps the draw sheet on the far side.

❑ 12. On the count of three, gently rolls resident toward self, turning resident as a unit.

❑ 13. Repositions resident comfortably.

❑ 14. Returns bed to appropriate level.

❑ 15. Places signaling device within resident's reach.

❑ 16. Washes hands.

❑ 17. Reports any changes in resident.

❑ 18. Documents procedure.

Comments:

❑ 6. Raises the head of bed to sitting position. Locks bed wheels.

❑ 7. Places one arm under resident's shoulder blades and the other arm under resident's thighs.

❑ 8. On the count of three, slowly turns resident into sitting position with legs dangling over side of bed.

❑ 9. Supports resident for 10 to 15 seconds. Checks for dizziness.

❑ 10. Assists resident to put on shoes or slippers.

❑ 11. Moves resident to edge of bed so feet are flat on floor.

❑ 12. Places signaling device within resident's reach.

❑ 13. Washes hands.

❑ 14. Reports any changes in resident.

❑ 15. Documents procedure.

Comments:

Assisting resident to sit up on side of bed

✓ Procedure Steps

❑ 1. Washes hands.

❑ 2. Identifies self to resident by name. Addresses resident by name.

❑ 3. Explains procedure to resident, speaking clearly, slowly, and directly, maintaining face-to-face contact whenever possible.

❑ 4. Provides for resident's privacy during procedure with curtain, screen, or door.

❑ 5. Adjusts bed height to lowest position.

Transferring a resident from bed to wheelchair

✓ Procedure Steps

❑ 1. Washes hands.

❑ 2. Identifies self to resident by name. Addresses resident by name.

❑ 3. Explains procedure to resident, speaking clearly, slowly, and directly, maintaining face-to-face contact whenever possible.

❑ 4. Provides for resident's privacy during procedure with curtain, screen, or door.

❑ 5. Positions wheelchair close to bed with arm of the wheelchair almost touching the bed. Places wheelchair on resident's stronger, or unaffected, side.

❑ 6. Folds up wheelchair footrests. Locks both wheels on wheelchair and bed.

❑ 7. Adjusts bed to its lowest level.

❑ 8. Assists resident to sitting position with feet flat on the floor.

❑ 9. Puts non-skid footwear on resident and securely fastens.

❑ 10. *With transfer (gait) belt*:

    a. Stands in front of resident.

    b. Stands with feet approximately 12 inches apart. Bends knees.

    c. Places belt around resident's waist. Grasps belt on both sides.

    Without transfer belt:

    a. Stands in front of resident.

    b. Stands with feet approximately 12 inches apart. Bends knees.

    c. Places arms around resident's torso under the arms.

❑ 11. Provides instructions to enable resident to assist in transfer.

❑ 12. With legs, braces resident's lower extremities to prevent slipping.

❑ 13. On signal, gradually assists resident to stand.

❑ 14. Assists resident to pivot to front of wheelchair with back of resident's legs against wheelchair.

❑ 15. Lowers resident into wheelchair.

❑ 16. Repositions resident with hips touching back of wheelchair and removes transfer belt, if used.

❑ 17. Positions resident's feet on footrests.

❑ 18. Places signaling device within resident's reach.

❑ 19. Washes hands.

❑ 20. Reports any changes in resident.

❑ 21. Documents procedure.

Comments:

SIX

Basic Nursing Skills

Admitting a resident

✓ **Procedure Steps**

❑ 1. Washes hands.

❑ 2. Identifies self to resident by name. Addresses resident by name.

❑ 3. Explains procedure to resident, speaking clearly, slowly, and directly, maintaining face-to-face contact whenever possible.

❑ 4. Provides for resident's privacy during procedure with curtain, screen, or door.

❑ 5. *If part of facility procedure, performs the following*:

    ❑ Takes resident's height and weight.

    ❑ Takes resident's vital signs.

    ❑ Obtains a urine specimen if required.

    ❑ Completes the paperwork, including an inventory of all the personal items.

    ❑ Assists resident to put personal items away.

    ❑ Provides fresh water.

□ 6. Orients resident to the room and bathroom. Explains how to work equipment.

□ 7. Introduces resident to roommate, other residents, and staff.

□ 8. Places signaling device within resident's reach.

□ 9. Washes hands.

□ 10. Documents procedure.

Comments:

Transferring a resident

✓ **Procedure Steps**

□ 1. Washes hands.

□ 2. Identifies self to resident by name. Addresses resident by name.

□ 3. Explains procedure to resident, speaking clearly, slowly, and directly, maintaining face-to-face contact whenever possible.

□ 4. Provides for resident's privacy during procedure with curtain, screen, or door.

□ 5. Collects the items to be transferred and takes them to the new location.

□ 6. Assists resident into the wheelchair or stretcher.

□ 7. Introduces new residents and staff.

□ 8. Assists resident to put personal items away.

□ 9. Makes sure that resident is comfortable. Places signaling device within resident's reach.

□ 10. Washes hands.

□ 11. Reports any changes in resident.

□ 12. Documents procedure.

Comments:

Discharging a resident

✓ **Procedure Steps**

□ 1. Washes hands.

□ 2. Identifies self to resident by name. Addresses resident by name.

□ 3. Explains procedure to resident, speaking clearly, slowly, and directly, maintaining face-to-face contact whenever possible.

□ 4. Provides for resident's privacy during procedure with curtain, screen, or door.

□ 5. Compares the checklist to the items there. If all items are there, asks resident to sign.

□ 6. Collects the items to be taken and takes them to pick-up area.

□ 7. Assists resident to dress and then into the wheelchair.

□ 8. Assists resident to say good-byes to the staff and residents.

□ 9. Transports resident to the pickup area. Assists resident into vehicle.

□ 10. Washes hands.

□ 11. Documents procedure.

Comments:

Taking and recording oral temperature

✓ **Procedure Steps**

□ 1. Washes hands.

❏ 2. Identifies self to resident by name. Addresses resident by name.

❏ 3. Explains procedure to resident, speaking clearly, slowly, and directly, maintaining face-to-face contact whenever possible.

❏ 4. Provides for resident's privacy during procedure with curtain, screen, or door.

Using a glass thermometer:

❏ 5. Holds thermometer by stem.

❏ 6. Shakes oral thermometer down to below the lowest number.

❏ 7. Puts on disposable sheath, if applicable. Inserts bulb end of oral thermometer into resident's mouth, under tongue and to one side.

❏ 8. Tells resident to hold oral thermometer in mouth with lips closed. Assists as necessary. Asks resident not to bite down or to talk.

❏ 9. Leaves oral thermometer in place for at least three minutes.

❏ 10. Removes the thermometer. Wipes with tissue from stem to bulb or removes sheath. Disposes of tissue or sheath.

❏ 11. Holds thermometer at eye level. Rotates until line appears. Reads and records temperature.

❏ 12. Cleans oral thermometer and/or returns it to container for used thermometers.

Using a digital thermometer:

❏ 5. Puts on disposable sheath.

❏ 6. Turns on thermometer and waits until "ready" sign appears.

❏ 7. Inserts end of digital thermometer into resident's mouth, under tongue and to one side.

❏ 8. Leaves in place until thermometer blinks or beeps.

❏ 9. Removes the thermometer.

❏ 10. Reads and records temperature on display screen.

❏ 11. Using a tissue, removes and disposes of sheath.

❏ 12. Replaces thermometer into case.

Using an electronic thermometer:

❏ 5. Removes probe from base unit.

❏ 6. Puts on probe cover.

❏ 7. Inserts end of electronic thermometer into resident's mouth, under tongue and to one side.

❏ 8. Leaves in place until tone or light signals temperature has been read.

❏ 9. Reads the temperature on the display screen.

❏ 10. Removes the probe. Presses the eject button to discard the cover.

❏ 11. Records temperature.

❏ 12. Returns the probe to the holder.

Final steps:

❏ 13. Places signaling device within resident's reach.

❏ 14. Washes hands.

❏ 15. Reports any changes in resident.

❏ 16. Documents procedure.

Comments:

Taking and recording axillary temperature

✓ **Procedure Steps**

❏ 1. Washes hands.

❑ 2. Identifies self to resident by name. Addresses resident by name.

❑ 3. Explains procedure to resident, speaking clearly, slowly, and directly, maintaining face-to-face contact whenever possible.

❑ 4. Provides for resident's privacy during procedure with curtain, screen, or door.

❑ 5. Rinses thermometer in cool water and dries with clean tissue.

❑ 6. Removes resident's arm from sleeve of gown. Wipes axillary area with tissues.

❑ 7. Holds thermometer at stem end and shakes down to below the lowest number.

❑ 8. Puts on disposable sheath, if applicable.

❑ 9. Places bulb end of thermometer in center of armpit and folds resident's arm over chest.

❑ 10. Holds in place for 10 minutes.

❑ 11. Removes the thermometer. Wipes with tissue from stem to bulb or removes sheath. Disposes of tissue or sheath.

❑ 12. Holds thermometer at eye level. Rotates until line appears. Reads and records temperature.

❑ 13. Cleans thermometer and/or returns it to container for used thermometers.

❑ 14. Puts resident's arm back into sleeve of gown.

❑ 15. Places signaling device within resident's reach.

❑ 16. Washes hands.

❑ 17. Reports any changes in resident.

❑ 18. Documents procedure.

Comments:

Taking and recording rectal temperature

✓ Procedure Steps

❑ 1. Washes hands.

❑ 2. Identifies self to resident by name. Addresses resident by name.

❑ 3. Explains procedure to resident, speaking clearly, slowly, and directly, maintaining face-to-face contact whenever possible.

❑ 4. Provides for resident's privacy during procedure with curtain, screen, or door.

❑ 5. Assists resident to side-lying position.

❑ 6. Folds back linens to expose rectal area.

❑ 7. Puts on gloves.

❑ 8. *Glass thermometer*: Holds thermometer by stem.

❑ *Digital thermometer*: Applies probe cover.

❑ 9. *Glass thermometer*: Shakes thermometer down to below the lowest number.

❑ 10. Applies small amount of lubricant to bulb or probe cover.

❑ 11. Gently inserts thermometer into rectum 1-1½ and a half inches.

❑ 12. Replaces sheet over buttocks.

❑ 13. *Glass thermometer*: Holds thermometer in place for at least three minutes. Holds onto the thermometer at all times while taking a rectal temperature.

❑ *Digital thermometer*: Holds thermometer in place until thermometer blinks or beeps. Holds onto the thermometer at all times while taking a rectal temperature.

❑ 14. Removes the thermometer. Wipes with tissue from stem to bulb or removes sheath. Disposes of tissue or sheath.

❑ 15. Reads thermometer and records temperature.

❑ 16. *Glass thermometer*: Washes thermometer and/or returns it to container for used thermometers.

❑   *Digital thermometer*: Throws away probe cover and returns thermometer to storage area.

❑ 17. Removes and disposes of gloves.

❑ 18. Assists resident to a position of safety and comfort.

❑ 19. Places signaling device within resident's reach.

❑ 20. Washes hands.

❑ 21. Reports any changes in resident.

❑ 22. Documents procedure.

Comments:

Taking and recording tympanic temperature

✓ **Procedure Steps**

❑ 1. Washes hands.

❑ 2. Identifies self to resident by name. Addresses resident by name.

❑ 3. Explains procedure to resident, speaking clearly, slowly, and directly, maintaining face-to-face contact whenever possible.

❑ 4. Provides for resident's privacy during procedure with curtain, screen, or door.

❑ 5. Puts a disposable sheath over earpiece of the thermometer.

❑ 6. Inserts the covered probe into the ear canal and presses the button.

❑ 7. Holds thermometer in place until thermometer blinks or beeps.

❑ 8. Reads and records temperature.

❑ 9. Disposes of sheath. Returns thermometer to storage area.

❑ 10. Places signaling device within resident's reach.

❑ 11. Washes hands.

❑ 12. Reports any changes in resident.

❑ 13. Documents procedure.

Comments:

Taking and recording radial pulse, and counting and recording respirations

✓ **Procedure Steps**

❑ 1. Washes hands.

❑ 2. Identifies self to resident by name. Addresses resident by name.

❑ 3. Explains procedure to resident, speaking clearly, slowly, and directly, maintaining face-to-face contact whenever possible.

❑ 4. Provides for resident's privacy during procedure with curtain, screen, or door.

❑ 5. Places fingertips on thumb side of resident's wrist to locate pulse.

❑ 6. Counts beats for one full minute.

❏ 7. Keeping fingertips on resident's wrist, counts respirations for one full minute.

❏ 8. Records pulse and respiration rate.

❏ 9. Places signaling device within resident's reach.

❏ 10. Washes hands.

❏ 11. Reports any changes in resident to the nurse.

❏ 12. Documents procedure.

Comments:

Taking and recording blood pressure (two-step method)

✓ **Procedure Steps**

❏ 1. Washes hands.

❏ 2. Identifies self to resident by name. Addresses resident by name.

❏ 3. Explains procedure to resident, speaking clearly, slowly, and directly, maintaining face-to-face contact whenever possible.

❏ 4. Provides for resident's privacy during procedure with curtain, screen, or door.

❏ 5. Positions resident's arm with palm up. The arm should be level with the heart.

❏ 6. With the valve open, squeezes the cuff to make sure it is completely deflated.

❏ 7. Places blood pressure cuff snugly on resident's upper arm, with the center of the cuff placed over the brachial artery (1-1½ inches above the elbow toward inside of elbow).

❏ 8. Locates the radial (wrist) pulse with fingertips.

❏ 9. Closes the valve (clockwise) until it stops. Inflates cuff, watching gauge.

❏ 10. Stops inflating cuff when pulse is no longer felt. Notes the reading. The number is an estimate of the systolic pressure.

❏ 11. Opens the valve to deflate cuff completely.

❏ 12. Writes down the systolic reading.

❏ 13. Wipes diaphragm and earpieces of stethoscope with alcohol wipes.

❏ 14. Locates brachial pulse with fingertips.

❏ 15. Places earpieces of stethoscope in ears.

❏ 16. Places diaphragm of stethoscope over brachial artery.

❏ 17. Closes the valve (clockwise) until it stops. Does not tighten it.

❏ 18. Inflates cuff to 30 mm Hg above the estimated systolic pressure.

❏ 19. Opens the valve slightly with thumb and index finger. Deflates cuff slowly.

❏ 20. Watches gauge and listens for sound of pulse.

❏ 21. Remembers the reading at which the first clear pulse sound is heard. This is the systolic pressure.

❏ 22. Continues listening for a change or muffling of pulse sound. The point of a change or the point the sound disappears is the diastolic pressure. Remembers this reading.

❏ 23. Opens the valve to deflate cuff completely. Removes cuff.

❏ 24. Records both systolic and diastolic pressures.

☐ 25. Wipes diaphragm and earpieces of stethoscope with alcohol. Stores equipment.

☐ 26. Places signaling device within resident's reach.

☐ 27. Washes hands.

☐ 28. Reports any changes in resident.

☐ 29. Documents procedure.

Comments:

Measuring and recording weight of an ambulatory resident

✓ **Procedure Steps**

☐ 1. Washes hands.

☐ 2. Identifies self to resident by name. Addresses resident by name.

☐ 3. Explains procedure to resident, speaking clearly, slowly, and directly, maintaining face-to-face contact whenever possible.

☐ 4. Provides for resident's privacy during procedure with curtain, screen, or door.

☐ 5. Starts with scale balanced at zero before weighing resident.

☐ 6. Assists resident to step onto the center of the scale.

☐ 7. Determines resident's weight.

☐ 8. Assists resident off scale before recording weight.

☐ 9. Records weight.

☐ 10. Places signaling device within resident's reach.

☐ 11. Washes hands.

☐ 12. Reports any changes in resident.

☐ 13. Documents procedure.

Comments:

Measuring and recording height of an ambulatory resident

✓ **Procedure Steps**

☐ 1. Washes hands.

☐ 2. Identifies self to resident by name. Addresses resident by name.

☐ 3. Explains procedure to resident, speaking clearly, slowly, and directly, maintaining face-to-face contact whenever possible.

☐ 4. Provides for resident's privacy during procedure with curtain, screen, or door.

☐ 5. Assists resident to step onto scale.

☐ 6. Asks resident to stand straight. Assists as needed.

☐ 7. Pulls up measuring rod from back of scale. Gently lowers measuring rod until it rests flat on resident's head.

☐ 8. Determines resident's height.

☐ 9. Assists resident off scale before recording height.

☐ 10. Records height.

☐ 11. Places signaling device within resident's reach.

☐ 12. Washes hands.

☐ 13. Reports any changes in resident.

☐ 14. Documents procedure.

Comments:

Measuring and recording urinary output

✓ **Procedure Steps**

❑ 1. Washes hands.

❑ 2. Puts on gloves before handling bedpan/urinal.

❑ 3. Pours the contents of the bedpan or urinal into measuring container without spilling or splashing any of the urine.

❑ 4. Measures the amount of urine while keeping container level.

❑ 5. After measuring urine, empties contents of measuring container into toilet without splashing.

❑ 6. Rinses measuring container and pours rinse water into toilet.

❑ 7. Rinses bedpan/urinal and pours rinse water into toilet.

❑ 8. Returns bedpan/urinal and measuring container to proper storage.

❑ 9. Removes and disposes of gloves.

❑ 10. Washes hands before recording output.

❑ 11. Records contents of container in output column on sheet.

❑ 12. Report any changes in resident.

Comments:

Providing catheter care

✓ **Procedure Steps**

❑ 1. Washes hands.

❑ 2. Identifies self to resident by name. Addresses resident by name.

❑ 3. Explains procedure to resident, speaking clearly, slowly, and directly, maintaining face-to-face contact whenever possible.

❑ 4. Provides for resident's privacy during procedure with curtain, screen, or door.

❑ 5. Adjusts bed to a safe working level.

❑ 6. Lowers head of bed. Positions resident lying flat on her back. Raises the side rail farthest from self.

❑ 7. Removes or folds back top bedding, keeping resident covered with bath blanket.

❑ 8. Tests water temperature with thermometer or wrist. Water temperature should be 105° to 109° F. Has resident check water temperature. Adjusts if necessary.

❑ 9. Puts on gloves.

❑ 10. Places clean protective pad under buttocks.

❑ 11. Exposes only the area necessary to clean the catheter.

❑ 12. Places towel or pad under catheter tubing before washing.

❑ 13. Applies soap to wet washcloth.

❑ 14. Holds catheter near meatus to avoid tugging the catheter.

❑ 15. Cleans at least four inches of catheter nearest meatus. Moves in only one direction, away from meatus. Uses a clean area of the cloth for each stroke.

❑ 16. Rinses at least four inches of catheter nearest meatus. Moves in only one direction, away from meatus. Uses a clean area of the cloth for each stroke.

❑ 17. Disposes of linen in proper containers.

❏ 18. Empties, rinses, and wipes basin and returns to proper storage.

❏ 19. Removes and disposes of gloves.

❏ 20. Returns bed to appropriate level. Puts signaling device within resident's reach.

❏ 21. Places soiled clothing and linens in appropriate containers.

❏ 22. Washes hands.

❏ 23. Reports any changes in resident.

❏ 24. Documents procedure.

Comments:

Collecting a clean catch (mid-stream) urine specimen

✓ **Procedure Steps**

❏ 1. Washes hands.

❏ 2. Identifies self to resident by name. Addresses resident by name.

❏ 3. Explains procedure to resident, speaking clearly, slowly, and directly, maintaining face-to-face contact whenever possible.

❏ 4. Provides for resident's privacy during procedure with curtain, screen, or door.

❏ 5. Puts on gloves.

❏ 6. Opens the specimen kit. Does not touch the inside of the container or the inside of the lid.

❏ 7. Using the towelettes or gauze and cleansing solution, cleans the area around the urethra. For females, separates the labia and wipes from front to back along one side. Discards towelette/gauze. With a new towelette or gauze, wipes from front to back along the other labia. Using a new towelette or gauze, wipes down the middle.

❏ For males, cleans the head of the penis using circular motions with the towelettes or gauze. Cleans thoroughly, changing towelettes/gauze after each circular motion and discarding after use. If the man is uncircumcised, pulls back the foreskin of the penis before cleaning and holds it back during urination. Makes sure it is pulled back down after collecting the specimen.

❏ 8. Asks resident to urinate into the bedpan, urinal, or toilet, and to stop before urination is complete.

❏ 9. Places the container under the urine stream and has resident start urinating again. Fills the container at least half full. Has resident finish urinating in bedpan, urinal, or toilet.

❏ 10. Covers the urine container with its lid. Wipes off the outside with a paper towel.

❏ 11. Places the container in a plastic bag.

❏ 12. If using a bedpan or urinal, discards extra urine. Rinses and cleans equipment, and stores.

❏ 13. Removes and disposes of gloves. Washes hands. Helps resident wash hands.

❏ 14. Completes the label for the container with resident's name, address, the date, and time.

❏ 15. Places signaling device within resident's reach.

❏ 16. Washes hands.

❏ 17. Reports any changes in resident.

❏ 18. Documents procedure. Notes amount and characteristics of urine.

Comments:

Collecting a stool specimen

✓ **Procedure Steps**

❏ 1. Washes hands.

❏ 2. Identifies self to resident by name. Addresses resident by name.

❏ 3. Explains procedure to resident, speaking clearly, slowly, and directly, maintaining face-to-face contact whenever possible.

❏ 4. Provides for resident's privacy during procedure with curtain, screen, or door.

❏ 5. Puts on gloves.

❏ 6. When resident is ready to move bowels, asks him not to urinate at the same time and not to put toilet paper in with the sample. Provides a plastic bag to discard toilet paper separately.

❏ 7. Fits specimen pan to toilet or commode, or provides resident with bedpan. Leaves the room and asks resident to signal when he is finished with the bowel movement. Makes sure call light is within resident's reach.

❏ 8. After the bowel movement, assists as necessary with perineal care. Helps resident wash his or her hands. Makes resident comfortable. Removes gloves.

❏ 9. Washes hands again.

❏ 10. Puts on clean gloves.

❏ 11. Using the two tongue blades, takes about two tablespoons of stool and puts it in the container. Covers it tightly.

❏ 12. Wraps the tongue blades in toilet paper and throws them away. Empties the bedpan or container into the toilet. Cleans and stores the equipment.

❏ 13. Completes the label for the container with resident's name, address, the date, and time. Bags the specimen.

❏ 14. Removes and disposes of gloves.

❏ 15. Places signaling device within resident's reach.

❏ 16. Washes hands.

❏ 17. Reports any changes in resident.

❏ 18. Documents procedure. Note amount and characteristics of stool.

Comments:

Making an occupied bed

✓ **Procedure Steps**

❏ 1. Washes hands.

❏ 2. Identifies self to resident by name. Addresses resident by name.

❏ 3. Explains procedure to resident, speaking clearly, slowly, and directly, maintaining face-to-face contact whenever possible.

❏ 4. Provides for resident's privacy during procedure with curtain, screen, or door.

❏ 5. Places clean linen on clean surface within reach.

❏ 6. Adjusts bed to a safe working level. Lowers head of bed before moving resident.

❏ 7. Puts on gloves if linens are soiled with body fluids.

❏ 8. Loosens top linen from the end of the bed or working side.

❑ 9. Raises side rail on far side of bed. Assists resident to turn onto side, moving away from self toward raised side rail.

❑ 10. Loosens bottom soiled linen on working side.

❑ 11. Rolls bottom soiled linen toward resident tucking it snugly against resident's back.

❑ 12. Places and tucks in clean bottom linen, finishing with bottom sheet free of wrinkles. Makes hospital corners to keep bottom sheet wrinkle-free.

❑ 13. Assists resident to turn onto clean bottom sheet. Raises side rail nearest self.

❑ 14. Moves to other side of bed and lowers side rail.

❑ 15. Turns resident away from self toward side rail.

❑ 16. Loosens soiled linen. Rolls linen from head to foot of bed. Avoids contact with skin or clothes. Places it in a hamper/bag, at foot of the bed, or in a chair.

❑ 17. Pulls and tucks in clean bottom linen, finishing with bottom sheet free of wrinkles.

❑ 18. Places resident on his back. Raises side rail.

❑ 19. Removes pillow. Changes pillowcase. Places pillow under resident's head with open end away from door.

❑ 20. Covers resident with clean top sheet. Removes soiled top sheet.

❑ 21. Finishes with the clean linen anchored and centered.

❑ 22. Unfolds blanket over top sheet.

❑ 23. Tucks top linens under foot of mattress and makes hospital corners.

❑ 24. Loosens top linens over resident's feet.

❑ 25. Returns bed to appropriate level. Puts signaling device within resident's reach.

❑ 26. Disposes of soiled linen in the soiled linen container.

❑ 27. Removes gloves if worn.

❑ 28. Washes hands.

❑ 29. Reports any changes in resident.

❑ 30. Documents procedure.

Comments:

Making an unoccupied bed

✓ Procedure Steps

❑ 1. Washes hands.

❑ 2. Places clean linen on clean surface within reach.

❑ 3. Adjusts bed to a safe working level. Puts bed in flattest position.

❑ 4. Puts on gloves if linens are soiled with body fluids.

❑ 5. Loosens soiled linen. Rolls soiled linen (soiled side inside) from head to foot of bed. Avoids contact with skin or clothes. Places it in a hamper/bag, at foot of the bed, or in chair.

❑ 6. Pulls and tucks in clean bottom linen, finishing with bottom sheet free of wrinkles. Makes hospital corners to keep bottom sheet wrinkle-free.

❑ 7. Applies top linen. Finishes with clean linen anchored and centered.

❑ 8. Unfolds blanket over top sheet.

❑ 9. Tucks top linens under foot of mattress and makes hospital corners.

❑ 10. Replaces pillowcase. Places pillow under resident's head at head of the bed with open end away from door.

❑ 11. Returns bed to appropriate level.

❑ 12. Disposes of soiled linen in the soiled linen container.

❑ 13. Removes gloves if worn.

❑ 14. Washes hands.

Comments:

Changing a dry dressing using non-sterile technique

✓ Procedure Steps

❑ 1. Washes hands.

❑ 2. Identifies self to resident by name. Addresses resident by name.

❑ 3. Explains procedure to resident, speaking clearly, slowly, and directly, maintaining face-to-face contact whenever possible.

❑ 4. Provides for resident's privacy during procedure with curtain, screen, or door.

❑ 5. Cuts pieces of tape long enough to secure the dressing. Hangs tape on the edge of a table within reach. Opens four-inch gauze square package without touching gauze. Places the opened package on a flat surface.

❑ 6. Puts on gloves.

❑ 7. Removes soiled dressing by gently peeling tape toward the wound. Lifts dressing off the wound. Does not drag it over wound. Observes dressing for any odor. Notes color of the wound. Disposes of used dressing in proper container. Removes and disposes of gloves.

❑ 8. Puts on new gloves. Touching only outer edges of new four-inch gauze, removes it from package. Applies it to wound. Tapes gauze in place. Secures it firmly.

❑ 9. Removes and disposes of gloves properly.

❑ 10. Places signaling device within resident's reach.

❑ 11. Washes hands.

❑ 12. Reports any changes in resident.

❑ 13. Documents procedure.

Comments:

SEVEN
Nutrition and Hydration

Serving fresh water

✓ Procedure Steps

❑ 1. Washes hands.

❑ 2. Identifies self to resident by name. Addresses resident by name.

❑ 3. Scoops ice into water pitcher. Adds fresh water.

❑ 4. Uses and stores ice scoop properly.

❑ 5. Takes pitcher of ice water to resident.

❑ 6. Pours glass of water for resident and leaves pitcher and glass at the bedside.

❑ 7. Makes sure that pitcher and glass are

light enough for resident to lift. Leaves a straw if resident desires.

❏ 8. Places signaling device within resident's reach.

❏ 9. Washes hands.

Comments:

Feeding a resident who cannot feed self

✓ Procedure Steps

❏ 1. Washes hands.

❏ 2. Identifies self to resident by name. Addresses resident by name.

❏ 3. Explains procedure to resident, speaking clearly, slowly, and directly, maintaining face-to-face contact whenever possible.

❏ 4. Assists resident to wash hands.

❏ 5. Before feeding resident, ensures resident is in an upright sitting position.

❏ 6. Verifies that resident has received the tray prepared for him/her.

❏ 7. Assists resident to put on clothing protector, if desired.

❏ 8. Sits at resident's eye level.

❏ 9. Offers drink of beverage. Alternates types of food offered, allowing for resident's preferences.

❏ 10. Offers the food in bite-sized pieces.

❏ 11. Makes sure resident's mouth is empty before next bite of food or sip of beverage.

❏ 12. Offers beverage to resident throughout the meal.

❏ 13. Talks with resident during meal.

❏ 14. Wipes food from resident's mouth and hands as necessary during the meal. Wipes again at the end of the meal.

❏ 15. Removes clothing protector if used. Disposes of in proper container.

❏ 16. Places signaling device within resident's reach.

❏ 17. Removes food tray. Checks for eyeglasses, dentures, or any personal items.

❏ 18. Washes hands.

❏ 19. Reports any changes in resident.

❏ 20. Documents procedure.

Comments:

EIGHT

Common, Chronic, and Acute Conditions

Putting a knee-high elastic stocking on resident

✓ Procedure Steps

❏ 1. Washes hands.

❏ 2. Identifies self to resident by name. Addresses resident by name.

❏ 3. Explains procedure to resident, speaking clearly, slowly, and directly, maintaining face-to-face contact whenever possible.

❏ 4. Provides for resident's privacy during procedure with curtain, screen, or door.

❏ 5. Turns stocking inside-out at least to heel area.

❏ 6. Gently places foot of stocking over toes, foot, and heel.

❏ 7. Gently pulls top of stocking over foot, heel, and leg.

❏ 8. Makes sure there are no twists or wrinkles in stocking after it is applied.

❏ 9. Places signaling device within resident's reach.

❏ 10. Washes hands.

❏ 11. Reports any changes in resident.

❏ 12. Documents procedure.

Comments:

Caring for an ostomy

✓ **Procedure Steps**

❏ 1. Washes hands.

❏ 2. Identifies self to resident by name. Addresses resident by name.

❏ 3. Explains procedure to resident, speaking clearly, slowly, and directly, maintaining face-to-face contact whenever possible.

❏ 4. Provides for resident's privacy during procedure with curtain, screen, or door.

❏ 5. Adjusts bed to a safe working level.

❏ 6. Places protective sheet under resident. Covers resident with a bath blanket. Pulls down the top sheet and blankets. Only exposes ostomy site. Offers resident a towel to keep clothing dry.

❏ 7. Puts on gloves.

❏ 8. Removes ostomy bag carefully. Places it in plastic bag. Notes the color, odor, consistency, and amount of stool in the bag.

❏ 9. Wipes the area around the stoma with toilet paper. Discards paper in plastic bag.

❏ 10. Using a washcloth and warm soapy water, washes the area around the stoma. Pats dry with another towel. Applies cream as ordered.

❏ 11. Places the clean ostomy appliance on resident. Makes sure the bottom of the bag is clamped.

❏ 12. Removes disposable bed protector and discards. Places soiled linens in appropriate containers.

❏ 13. Removes bag and bedpan. Discards bag in proper container. Empties contents of bedpan into toilet.

❏ 14. Cleans bedpan, pouring rinse water into toilet. Returns to proper storage.

❏ 15. Removes and disposes of gloves properly.

❏ 16. Returns bed to appropriate level. Places signaling device within resident's reach.

❏ 17. Washes hands.

❏ 18. Reports any changes in resident.

❏ 19. Documents procedure.

Comments:

NINE

Rehabilitation and Restorative Services

Assisting a resident to ambulate

✓ **Procedure Steps**

❑ 1. Washes hands.

❑ 2. Identifies self to resident by name. Addresses resident by name.

❑ 3. Explains procedure to resident, speaking clearly, slowly, and directly, maintaining face-to-face contact whenever possible.

❑ 4. Provides for resident's privacy during procedure with curtain, screen, or door.

❑ 5. Before ambulating, puts on and properly fastens non-skid footwear on resident.

❑ 6. Adjusts bed to a safe working level.

❑ 7. Stands in front of and faces resident.

❑ 8. Braces resident's lower extremities. Bends knees. Places one foot between resident's knees.

❑ 9. *With transfer (gait) belt*: Places belt around resident's waist and grasps the belt, while assisting resident to stand.

❑ *Without transfer belt*: Places arms around resident's torso under resident's armpits, while assisting resident to stand.

❑ 10. *With transfer belt*: Walks slightly behind and to one side of resident for the full distance, while holding onto the transfer belt.

❑ *Without transfer belt*: Walks slightly behind and to one side of resident for the full distance, with arm supporting resident's back.

❑ 11. After ambulation, removes transfer belt if used. Assists resident to a comfortable position.

❑ 12. Returns bed to appropriate level.

❑ 13. Places signaling device within resident's reach.

❑ 14. Washes hands.

❑ 15. Reports any changes in resident.

❑ 16. Documents procedure.

Comments:

Assisting with ambulation for a resident using a cane, walker, or crutches

✓ **Procedure Steps**

❑ 1. Washes hands.

❑ 2. Identifies self to resident by name. Addresses resident by name.

❑ 3. Explains procedure to resident, speaking clearly, slowly, and directly, maintaining face-to-face contact whenever possible.

❑ 4. Provides for resident's privacy during procedure with curtain, screen, or door.

❑ 5. Before ambulating, puts on and properly fastens non-skid footwear on resident.

❑ 6. Adjusts bed to a safe working level.

❑ 7. Stands in front of and faces resident.

❑ 8. Braces resident's lower extremities. Bends knees. Places one foot between resident's knees.

❑ 9. Places transfer belt around resident's

waist and grasps the belt, while assisting resident to stand.

❑ 10. Assists as necessary with ambulation with cane, walker, or crutches.

❑ 11. Walks slightly behind and to one side of resident. Holds the transfer belt if one is used.

❑ 12. Watches for obstacles in resident's path. Encourages resident to look ahead, rather than down at his or her feet.

❑ 13. Encourages resident to rest if fatigued. Lets resident set the pace.

❑ 14. After ambulation, removes transfer belt. Assists resident to a position of comfort and safety.

❑ 15. Returns bed to appropriate level.

❑ 16. Places signaling device within resident's reach.

❑ 17. Washes hands.

❑ 18. Reports any changes in resident.

❑ 19. Documents procedure.

Comments:

Assisting with passive range of motion (PROM) exercises

✓ **Procedure Steps**

❑ 1. Washes hands.

❑ 2. Identifies self to resident by name. Addresses resident by name.

❑ 3. Explains procedure to resident, speaking clearly, slowly, and directly, maintaining face-to-face contact whenever possible.

❑ 4. Provides for resident's privacy during procedure with curtain, screen, or door.

❑ 5. Adjusts bed to a safe working level.

❑ 6. Positions resident lying supine—flat on his or her back—on the bed. Positions body in good alignment.

❑ 7. While supporting the limbs, moves all joints gently, slowly, and smoothly through the range of motion to the point of resistance. Stops exercises if any pain occurs.

❑ 8. Shoulder. Performs the following exercises:

    ❑ forward flexion

    ❑ extension

    ❑ abduction

    ❑ adduction

    ❑ internal rotation

    ❑ external rotation

❑ 9. Elbow. Performs the following exercises:

    ❑ flexion

    ❑ extension

    ❑ pronation

    ❑ supination

❑ 10. Wrist. Performs the following exercises:

    ❑ flexion

    ❑ extension

    ❑ radial flexion

    ❑ ulnar flexion

❑ 11. Thumb. Performs the following exercises:

    ❑ abduction

    ❑ adduction

    ❑ opposition

    ❑ flexion

    ❑ extension

Name: _____

❏ 12. Fingers. Performs the following
      exercises:

    ❏   flexion

    ❏   extension

    ❏   abduction

    ❏   adduction

❏ 13. Hip. Performs the following exercises:

    ❏   abduction

    ❏   adduction

    ❏   internal rotation

    ❏   external rotation

❏ 14. Knees. Performs the following
      exercises:

    ❏   flexion

    ❏   extension

❏ 15. Ankles. Performs the following
      exercises:

    ❏   dorsiflexion

    ❏   plantar flexion

    ❏   supination

    ❏   pronation

❏ 16. Toes. Performs the following
      exercises:

    ❏   flexion and extension

    ❏   abduction

❏ 17. Returns bed to appropriate level.

❏ 18. Places signaling device within resi-
      dent's reach.

❏ 19. Washes hands.

❏ 20. Reports any changes in resident.

❏ 21. Documents procedure.

Comments:

PRACTICE EXAM

The Nursing Assistant's Handbook

Taking an Exam

Your physical condition affects your mental abilities. Watch what you eat and drink before taking a test and get plenty of rest. On the day of the exam, eat a power breakfast. It's hard to think if your stomach is growling. Also, being in good physical shape allows for more blood to get to your brain. A person who gets regular physical exercise has a body and mind that uses its oxygen more effectively than someone completely out of shape. Even exercising a few days before a test can make a noticeable difference in your thinking powers.

When taking the exam, listen carefully to any instructions given. Be sure to read the directions. When taking a multiple choice test, first eliminate answers you know are wrong. Since your first choice is usually correct, don't change your answers unless you are sure of the correction.

Don't spend too much time on any one question. If you do not understand it, move on and come back if time allows. Remember to leave that question blank on your answer sheet! Be careful to answer the next question in the proper space.

For the skills portion of the exam, review the procedures in the book. Pay special attention to the alerts that follow the procedure. These are commonly missed steps on the exams.

Remember that being nervous is natural. Most people get nervous before and during a test. A little stress can actually help you focus and make you more alert. A few deep breaths can help calm you down. Try it.

Most importantly, believe in yourself. You can do it!

1. When a resident refuses to let the nursing assistant take her blood pressure, the nursing assistant should:

   a. respect the resident's wishes

   b. take the resident's blood pressure anyway

   c. tell the resident that if she does this, she will get dessert later

   d. report this to the nurse

2. A nursing assistant may share a resident's medical information with which of the following?

   a. the resident's friends

   b. other members of the healthcare team

   c. the nursing assistant's friends

   d. the resident's roommate

3. To best communicate with a resident who has a hearing impairment, the nursing assistant should:

   a. use short sentences and simple words

   b. shout

   c. approach the resident from behind

   d. raise the pitch of her voice

4. Which of the following is NOT an example of abuse or neglect?

   a. assisting a resident to make a complaint

   b. not answering a resident's call light

   c. leaving a resident in a soiled bed

   d. threatening to hit a resident

5. An ombudsman is a person who:

   a. is in charge of the facility

   b. teaches nursing assistants how to perform ROM exercises

   c. is a legal advocate for residents and helps protect their rights

   d. creates special diets for residents

6. To best respond to a resident with Alzheimer's disease who is repeating a question over and over again, the nursing assistant should:

   a. answer questions each time they are asked, using the same words

   b. try to silence the resident

   c. tell the resident to stop

   d. explain to the resident that he just asked that question

7. Regarding a resident's toenails, a nursing assistant should:

   a. never cut them

   b. cut them when the resident requests it

   c. cut them daily

   d. file them into rounded edges

8. When providing care, the nursing assistant should:

   a. make sure the resident doesn't talk

   b. provide privacy for the resident

   c. tell the resident about other resident's conditions

   d. discuss personal problems

9. Generally, the last sense to leave a dying resident is the:

   a. sense of sight

   b. sense of taste

   c. sense of smell

   d. sense of hearing

10. Which temperature is considered the most accurate?

    a. rectal

    b. oral

    c. axillary

    d. tympanic

11. How should a standard bedpan be positioned?

    a. according to the resident's preference

    b. wider end aligned with resident's buttocks

    c. smaller end aligned with resident's buttocks

    d. smaller end facing the resident's head

12. A resident tells a nursing assistant that she is scared of dying. How should the nursing assistant respond?

    a. Reply, "You should attend church services more often. Then you won't be so afraid."

    b. Listen quietly and ask questions when appropriate.

    c. Laugh and tell the resident "You won't be going anywhere soon."

    d. Reply, "You need to start taking new medication."

13. To prevent dehydration a nursing assistant should:

   a. discourage fluids before bedtime

   b. withhold fluids so the resident will be really thirsty

   c. offer fresh water and other fluids often

   d. wake the resident during the night to offer fluids

14. When giving perineal care to a female resident, a nursing assistant should:

   a. wipe from front to back

   b. wipe from back to front

   c. use the same section of the washcloth for cleaning each part

   d. wash the anal area before the perineal area

15. If a nursing assistant sees a resident masturbating, the nursing assistant should:

   a. run to the charge nurse and ask her what to do

   b. provide privacy for the resident

   c. tell the resident that he shouldn't be doing that

   d. laugh and tell the other nursing assistants what happened

16. Range of motion exercises move each muscle and joint. The purpose of these exercises includes all of the following EXCEPT:

   a. to increase circulation

   b. to improve strength

   c. to cause pain

   d. to prevent contractures

17. A nursing assistant must wear gloves when:

   a. combing a resident's hair

   b. feeding a resident

   c. performing oral care

   d. performing range of motion exercises

18. To best communicate with a resident who has a vision impairment, the nursing assistant should:

   a. rearrange furniture without telling the resident

   b. identify herself when she enters the room

   c. keep the lighting low at all times

   d. touch the resident before identifying herself

19. The first sign of skin breakdown is:

   a. coolness

   b. bleeding

   c. discoloration

   d. numbness

20. Which one of the following statements is true about the normal aging process and late adulthood (65 years and older)?

   a. People become helpless and lonely.

   b. People become incontinent.

   c. People develop Alzheimer's disease.

   d. People are generally active and engaged.

21. Clean bed linens promote:

   a. proper rest and sleep

   b. infection and disease

   c. pressure sores

   d. poor circulation

22. The Heimlich maneuver uses abdominal thrusts to:

    a. stop bleeding

    b. remove blockage from an airway

    c. reduce the risk of falls

    d. stop a heart attack

23. All of the following are ways to prevent weight loss EXCEPT:

    a. Helping residents who have trouble feeding themselves

    b. Hurrying residents through meals

    c. Providing oral care before and after meals

    d. Honoring food likes and dislikes

24. Using proper body mechanics includes all of the following EXCEPT:

    a. bending knees while lifting

    b. standing with feet shoulder-length apart while lifting

    c. keeping an object close to the body after lifting it

    d. twisting at the waist when moving an object

25. What would be the best way for a nursing assistant to promote a resident's independence and dignity during bowel or bladder retraining?

    a. rushing the resident

    b. providing privacy for elimination

    c. criticizing a resident when he has a setback

    d. withholding fluids

26. A resident tells a nursing assistant that he wants to wear his gray sweater. The nursing assistant should:

    a. tell him that she has already picked out his clothes for the day

    b. tell him "okay" and assist him in getting dressed

    c. tell him that his gray sweater does not match his pants and ask him to pick something else

    d. tell him that she likes his blue sweater better

27. A nursing assistant should wash her hands:

    a. before a procedure

    b. before and after a procedure

    c. after a procedure

    d. while wearing gloves

28. How should soiled bed linen be handled?

    a. by carrying them away from the nursing assistant's body

    b. by shaking them in the air before disposing of them

    c. by taking them into another resident's room

    d. by taking them into the cafeteria

29. Residents have all of the following rights EXCEPT:

    a. the right to refuse treatment

    b. the right to voice complaints

    c. the right to make personal choices, such as what to wear and how to spend their time

    d. the right to be abused by nursing assistants if they're being combative

30. One safety device that helps transfer residents is called a:

    a. waist restraint

    b. a Posey vest

    c. a transfer or gait belt

    d. a geriatric chair

31. When cleaning a mercury glass thermometer, a nursing assistant should:

    a. use hot water

    b. use bleach

    c. use shampoo

    d. use cool water

32. A nursing assistant should encourage a resident's independence and self-care because they:

    a. promote body function

    b. decrease blood flow

    c. lower self-esteem

    d. decrease the ability to sleep and rest

33. A restraint can be applied:

    a. when a resident is being rude

    b. when a nursing assistant does not have time to watch the resident

    c. with a doctor's order

    d. when a resident keeps pressing his call light

34. A nursing assisting can show she is listening carefully to a resident by:

    a. looking away when the resident talks

    b. changing the subject often

    c. rolling her eyes when the resident says something she doesn't agree with

    d. responding to the resident when it's appropriate

35. How many cubic centimeters equal one ounce?

    a. 40

    b. 30

    c. 60

    d. 20

36. With catheters it is important for a nursing assistant to remember that:

    a. tubing should be kinked

    b. perineal care does not need to be performed

    c. the drainage bag should be kept lower than the hips or the bladder

    d. the resident should lie on top of the tubing

37. When assisting a resident who has had a stroke, a nursing assistant should:

    a. do everything for the resident

    b. lead with the stronger side when transferring

    c. dress the stronger side first

    d. place food in the affected, or weaker, side of the mouth

38. Which stage of dying would it be if a resident insists that a mistake was made on his blood test and he's not really dying?

    a. denial

    b. bargaining

    c. acceptance

    d. depression

39. The process of restoring a person to the highest level of functioning is called:

    a. Positioning

    b. Rehabilitation

    c. Elimination

    d. Retention

40. A nursing assistant overhears other nursing assistants discussing a resident. One of them says that she doesn't like taking care of this resident because "he is rude and smells funny." The nursing assistant should:

   a. join in the conversation and tell the others her opinion of this resident

   b. not respond to the conversation and leave the area

   c. suggest to the nursing assistants that this isn't the place to have this discussion

   d. ask another resident's opinion of how she should respond

41. An oral temperature should NOT be taken on a resident who has eaten or drunk fluids in the last _____ minutes.

   a. 25-35

   b. 10-20

   c. 40-50

   d. 50-60

42. Which of the following statements about canes is true?

   a. Canes cannot help with balance.

   b. Canes are used for residents who cannot bear any weight.

   c. A straight cane can bear all of a resident's weight.

   d. A quad cane has four rubber-tipped feet.

43. A nursing assistant can assist residents with their spiritual needs by:

   a. trying to convince residents to change to the nursing assistant's religion

   b. listening to residents talk about their beliefs

   c. insisting residents participate in religious services

   d. expressing judgments about residents' religious groups

44. The best way for a nursing assistant to respond to a combative resident is to:

   a. hit the resident

   b. argue with the resident if what the resident is saying is wrong

   c. not to take it personally

   d. tell the resident he is behaving childishly

45. When a resident has a right-sided weakness, how should clothing be applied first?

   a. on the left side

   b. on the right side

   c. on whichever side is closer to the nursing assistant

   d. whatever side the resident prefers

46. A resident offers a nursing assistant a gift for being such a good nursing assistant. The nursing assistant should:

   a. politely refuse the gift

   b. politely accept the gift

   c. accept the gift but donate it to a homeless shelter

   d. tell the resident she'd really prefer money instead